HIJRAS, LOVERS, BROTHERS

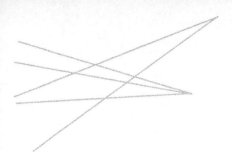

HIJRAS, LOVERS, BROTHERS

Surviving Sex and Poverty in Rural India

VAIBHAV SARIA

FORDHAM UNIVERSITY PRESS NEW YORK 2021

Awarded the Joseph W. Elder Prize in the Indian Social Sciences by the American Institute of Indian Studies and published with the Institute's generous support.

AIIS Publication Committee: Sarah Lamb, Co-Chair, Anand A. Yang, Co-Chair, Chanchal Dadlani, Diane Mines, Tulasi Srinivas, Tariq Thachil

Fordham University Press gratefully acknowledges financial assistance and support provided for the publication of this book by Simon Fraser University.

Library of Congress Cataloging-in-Publication Data

Names: Saria, Vaibhav, author.
Title: Hijras, lovers, brothers : surviving sex and poverty in rural India / Vaibhav Saria.
Description: New York : Fordham University Press, 2021. | Series: Thinking from elsewhere | Includes bibliographical references and index.
Identifiers: LCCN 2021005886 | ISBN 9780823294701 (hardback) | ISBN 9780823294718 (paperback) | ISBN 9780823294725 (epub)
Subjects: LCSH: Gender-nonconforming people—India—Social conditions. | Gender-nonconforming people—India—Economic conditions. | Rural poor—India.
Classification: LCC HQ73.85.I4 S27 2021 | DDC 306.76/8—dc23
LC record available at https://lccn.loc.gov/2021005886

Printed in the United States of America

23 22 21   5 4 3 2 1

First edition

To Aaron Goodfellow
with immeasurable admiration and gratitude

CONTENTS

HIJRAS, LOVERS, BROTHERS

INTRODUCTION

That Limpid Liquid within Young Men

One of my earliest memories is overhearing a conversation between my mother and my aunt regarding hijras. Hijras are now translated as "transgenders" or "trans women," but more on that in a bit. My aunt had asked my mother, "Where do 'they' come from?" after seeing them beg on the streets, and my mother replied, "They are born this way and when they come to bless the newborn baby, they check the genitals; if the baby is born like them then they take the baby away." I cannot tell you, dear reader, the sense of relief that this snippet of information inspired in my young self. This was in the mid-1990s, when I must have been six or seven years old, before the Internet had made the discourse surrounding sexual minorities more accessible. I knew by then that something was not right with me; I was born a certain "way"—not surprising, given the ordinary cruel teasing I was meted by everybody, every day. I knew at that moment that if I were kicked out by my family, or if I ran away, then I could seek shelter with hijras; they would take care of someone "born like them." Little did I know that, years later, hijras would not only help me survive but teach me how to thrive. Thus, this book seeks to describe the fullness of hijra lives in India. It documents the lessons I was taught on how to see, and how to receive the world, when everything seemed incomprehensibly cruel, as they often are for young trans people.

Hijras have been an enduring presence in the South Asian imagination—in myth, in ritual (particularly associated with rites of passage such as births and marriages), and in everyday life, often associated in stigmatized forms with begging and sex work. In more recent years hijras have been associated with a degree of political emergence as an explicitly moral presence in Indian electoral politics and with heightened vulnerability within global health terms, a high-risk population caught within the AIDS epidemic, sex work being one of the traditional hijra occupations.

This book recounts twenty-four months of fieldwork conducted between 2008 and 2019, including sixteen continuous months of living with a group of hijras in two of the poorest districts of India, Bhadrak and Kalahandi, in the state of Odisha in eastern India. Collecting alms on trains and street corners and otherwise participating in the everyday concerns of my interlocutors revealed not just a group of stigmatized or marginalized others, but rather a way of life composed of laughter, kinship, struggles, and desires.

In elaborating the hijra way of life, I hope to show how it troubles some commonly held concepts by which we read queerness, kinship, and the psyche. First, where queer theory has often cast the future in terms of negation or along an axis where the promise of "Western" liberalism faces its postcolonial critique, I seek to show the more ambivalent ways in which hijras face promise and futurity, through impossible longings, fratricidal kinship systems, economies ranging from property inheritance and begging, to tax shaming and semen, and the ways Hindu and Muslim myth and ritual alternate in hijra lives to reconstitute gender and temporality. In this book I address the hijra form of being as a mode of political theology that inhabits and exceeds the liberal political order.

Second, I seek to intervene in discussions within South Asian anthropology and kinship studies more broadly by drawing out the consistent and systematic parallel between hijras and asceticism as a "diagonal" relation to heteronormative social formations. In "World Renunciation in Indian Religions," Louis Dumont argued that "the dialogue between the householder and the ascetic might be seen as the secret animating Indian religions."[1] Bringing this insight and dialogue to bear on the study of hijras allows us to reinterpret the relation between margin and norm.

This book also seeks to intervene in psychoanalytic theory. Rather than recognizing a dichotomy between Western and Indian concepts of the psyche, I illustrate a series of displacements away from lack and negation and toward a picture of desire, gaps, and longings that include "phantom" babies, fratricidal siblings, and "unsafe" labors of love that are not fully legible either as death drive or as fullness. Finally, I seek to shift the terms with which we talk about a population perceived as high-risk in light of the AIDS epidemic in India. Rather than being cast only through the optic of precarity or resilience, hijras place themselves within broader questions of "living and dying in the contemporary world," as Clara Han and Veena Das have phrased it.[2]

TRANSLATING TRANS

Hijras are often translated as "transgenders" in the English media and in the legal discourse of India. Referring to hijras as transgenders and not trans women encapsulates complexities that haunt queer studies and anthropology. Hijras, with their long-documented history, are not a local or cultural instantiation of the global category of trans, and neither is this a new question of how to recognize in hijras some universal pattern. Hijras were referred to as "eunuchs" in much of colonial discourse and in English language dailies until quite recently. Hijras were and continue to be indexed as South Asia's "third gender," harkening to an impulse in the 1970s and 1980s to marshal evidence from all around the world and curate them in an encyclopedic fashion to make a case for the "nonbinary" and "fluid" nature of gender.[3] An earlier reiteration of the trope of universal sexual deviancy, albeit with different moral charges, was seen in the hypothesis of the Sotadic Zone. This hypothesis, put forward by Richard Burton during the mid-nineteenth century, was built on thinking about sexuality geographically, in climatic and constitutional terms, drawing from and contributing to the orientalist imagination.[4]

Against this background, hijras were included by the British Raj in the Indian Criminal Tribes Act of 1871, at the insistence of a member of the drafting committee, who believed that they were managers of "an organized system of sodomitical prostitution" and particularly unwilling to "adopt 'honest pursuits.'" The act prohibited hijras from appearing in public wearing female clothing, but the fact that hijras were also performers, actors, and theater artists made it difficult for the colonial police to effectively enact this criminalization.[5] Furthermore, at the end of the nineteenth century, with the annexation of various princely states—in the courts of which hijras had fairly respectable positions—hijras' claims to land and property (gifted by the royal family), along with the right to collect money from the exchequers of these principalities, were dissolved, resulting in an impoverished community by the time of independence.[6]

The most familiar and widely known word for trans women is "hijras," though the word is now so widely used disparagingly that hijra activists have recovered from Hindu mythology another word to refer to themselves: *kinnar*. This political project of renaming, using *kinnar*, has yet to reach the sites where I did my research, and has been received with suspicion by some activists, since it could possibly be an alibi to absorb hijras within ascendant right-wing Hindu nationalism. I use the word "hijra" throughout the book not only because my friends and informants used it but also because translating hijras as trans women would close questions, rather than open them. It would settle matters rather than raise them. Hijras can be translated as trans women with the caveat that we take "trans" to be an open-ended signifier to include "transgenders"; only then can we take this book as part of a growing scholarship on trans persons. In other words, the signifier "transgender" forces us to acknowledge the varied, plural, and at times contradictory careers of the word and modifier "trans" in different parts of the world.[7] Using the word "transgender" is a way to avoid using the word "hijra," since the word has been and continues to be used disparagingly by some people; it is a way of according respect, as seen in the text of Indian legal and parliamentary documents. The move to accord respect is part of a larger change in the relationship between the Indian state and hijras, a change that is predicated on the religious importance of hijras that the Hindu nationalist Indian state finds opportune to recognize.[8] The fact that citizenship is given cognizance because of religious importance rather than because of democratic ideals of equality, as has been the case with gay marriage in the Euro-American West, raises questions about the relationship of queerness to secular liberalism. Indeed, hijras and trans women do not have a simple corresponding relationship; the stakes for trans women to consider themselves hijras are different from hijras considering themselves as trans women. Trans women, by using the word, are signaling access to capital and discourse to which many hijras do not have access. They could also use the word to differentiate themselves from the form of life that hijras inhabit, such as begging, prostitution, and community membership, among others—all of which will be discussed in this book. Some hijras do identify themselves as trans women, especially those in urban centers who have been recruited by global health initiatives as local experts for HIV prevention, and thus it is the issue of class that determines who becomes familiar with the term, its meaning, discourse and claims, identity and currency.

The men I loved have aged well.
Some even married lookers.
Their women gave birth to sons
who resembled their mothers.

These men no longer call,
no knocking at my door—
no longer look for sustenance,
my shadow's wings and more.

Lost boys, they had their uses,
those men who always married—
said their say, paid their way
and then did their harm.

Still I should forgive them
since what will be will be—
boyfriends giving life to sons,
boyfriends, who once loved me.

—Frank McGuinness, "Boyfriends"

Lee Edelman's influential argument in *No Future: Queer Theory and the Death Drive* (2004) would reframe hijras in Lacanian terms as a subject that threatens to undo the symbolic, but more importantly as a subject who by resisting "the viability of the social . . . [insists] on the inextricability of such resistance from every social structure."[9] Edelman continues to argue for the paradoxical relation between the symbolic and the excess that it produces, the death drive; that is, between the futurism insisted on by reproductive heteronormativity and the future-annihilating queer. Leo Bersani raises the question of how not to have an investment in futurity in his blurb on the back cover of Edelman's book: "The paradoxical dignity of queerness would be its refusal to believe in a redemptive future, its embrace of the unintelligibility, even the inhumanity inherent in sexuality. Edelman's extraordinary text is so powerful that we could perhaps reproach him only for not spelling out the mode in which we might survive our necessary assent to his argument." Bersani's playful reproach is an entry point for anthropology to engage in the dialogue because, simply put, not everyone's experience of time sutures the past, present, and future in a manner that might give birth to futurity. In other words, not everybody experiences temporality as determined by secular liberalism, and given the religious meanings attached to hijras in India, the temporality that structures their lives borrows from longstanding histories and traditions of asceticism.

Thus, larger questions that are provoked by the antisocial thesis could be, How are futures imagined? How is the category conceived? Furthermore, the religious underpinnings of secular liberalism are not particular to hijras but have been a definitive characteristic of this concept in South Asia and indeed elsewhere, as scholars of "political theology" have shown.[10] In fact, this worlding of concepts is particularly sharp when we look at queer sexuality outside the Euro-American West, which carries religious and cultural significance, as opposed to its counterpart in the Christian West, which enjoys secular liberal citizenship. This worlding is one way in which anthropology gets "ethnographically detained" when it reveals different views of the world even when the same lens, such as liberalism, secularism, or religion, is applied.[11] Thus, while Edelman preaches a liberating cauterization of futurity, my gesture, following the hijras, in contrast, is to move diagonally to the linear unfolding of time. The implication of this gesture does not involve the denial of liberalism's existence outside "the West." Rather, it reveals that liberation for hijras is not from religion, as in a Christian context; rather, myths and religious texts are routes to engage the liberal democratic state in India. Such a formulation moves beyond the binary of whether gender/sexuality is a secular or a theological issue and asks more *how* it becomes secular and *how* it becomes a religious issue.

Even if it may be pointlessly provocative, consider this example: given that some children grow up to be men that hijras fuck, may one then not actively or passively ethically support the reproductive futurism of others? The anthropological truth that it takes a village to raise a child could be reformulated when viewed through Edelman's scintillatingly poisonous articulation of sexuality to read: you may help raise children to grow into men who might eventually become lovers of hijras in the future.[12] The following chapters show how hijras perform Edelman's edict not to participate in reproductive futurism to the extent that they are not signatories to children

6   *Introduction*

and contracts of lineages. But to the extent that they do participate in the various scenes of the social that erase the queer's trace while being sustained by that negation at the same time, they pose a complexly profound challenge to the simple command to not reproduce.

The subtraction of the child, moreover, would necessarily require from hijras a theological explanation—given that the child in the Hindu world also saves one's soul. The *sloka* (Sanskrit couplet) that is cited in several ancient texts, including the *Manusmriti*, has been translated by Patrick Olivelle as "The Self-Existent One himself has called him 'son' (*putra*) because he rescues (*tra*) his father from the hell named *Put*."[13] Robert Goldman's translation is more colloquial: "Since a son saves (*trayate*) his father from hell called *Put*, he was therefore declared to be 'put-tra' by Brahma himself."[14] The soul is the location through which we can qualify hijras' asceticism; this is a focal argument of Chapter 3. How one experiences, organizes, and marks time when one subtracts the "order of the child" when it is also the order of the symbolic is a concern for ascetics. Ascetics, or *sanyasis*, as Veena Das writes, represent the category of the asocial (in the sense that they are outside the domain of the family, kinship, and caste) and someone belonging to it who "can *force* God to establish a relation with him if his austerity is severe enough."[15]

Hijras' eroticism would follow Edelman's argument, which has been called the "antisocial thesis" in Queer Theory, and their asceticism would give them the place of the asocial, pace Das's analysis of the nexus of relations between the king, the brahman, and the sanyasi.[16] The instantiation of eroticism and asceticism within the figure of the hijra reminds us that there is a third function in the Hindu trimurti in addition to creating and destroying: that is preserving. Edelman's argument regarding what negativity does seem to me very much to fulfill the function of preserving.[17] The issue of asceticism becomes salient for this study because it offers a way to answer the question of what nonheteronormative temporality might look like—or, at least, what it does look like for hijras in rural Odisha. But before we move to the next section, I want to caution the reader to not read asceticism in narrow terms but instead see it as an instantiation of morality in the context of queer sexuality and poverty, just as Weber offers an alternate asceticism in his study of puritanism and capitalism.

At around four in the morning Damru and I were lolling about, unable to sleep, when Nandita returned from the highway and walked over to us after parking her cycle. She looked quite giddy, and I thought she was drunk. She showed me a used condom and between fits of laughter said, "I finally ate Saajan."[18] Swaying with joy and laughter, she proceeded to empty the contents of the condom into her mouth. She spat the semen back into the condom, laughed, and said, "Ah, seven months of thirst is finally quenched." I asked her why she spat it back into the condom instead of swallowing it, and she replied that she will put it in her mouth again and repeat it until it is all gone. "I want his smell in my mouth, so that I can smell him every time I breathe. It's like perfume, it makes me heady (*nasha*)." (*Nasha* translates and is used to describe drugs—and metaphorically, love—and their effect.) How are we to read this conflation of metaphors? Perfume is swallowed, water is spat out, and *nasha* is not inhaled but exhaled. The metaphor fuses several binaries—and this is where I begin discussing hijras' sexuality, which makes them historical figures of queerness as well as a population at risk for HIV.

Leo Bersani, in his study of *Madame Bovary*—another text famous for the fusion of metaphors—writes, "The natural inclination of Flaubertian desire is toward dangerous fusions; in other terms, desire leads to the nightmare of a loss of form."[19] I want to totter forth with this loss of form in Nandita's statement as I begin this study of desire predicated upon sexual transactions, like the one that occurred between Nandita and Saajan. Richard Halpern's analysis of a Shakespearean sonnet may help us reflect further on the metaphor:

> But if the image of perfume and glass is vastly ill-suited to its stated purpose of figuring sexual procreation, it is as more than one critic has noticed, perfectly suited to another, implied purpose: that of figuring *poetic* procreation. The diminutive, unchanging perfection of the perfume bottle thus represents not a baby but a sonnet. The glass womb is the male womb of Shakespearean verse, in which the young man's essence will be perpetuated, not as another living and therefore perishable blossom but rather as eternal though static lines of poetry.[20]

If perfuming the semen in the Shakespearean sonnet is a kind of procreation, what is it exactly that is being engendered in Nandita's womb? I should hasten to point out that Nandita, in a way, conflates her mouth and her rectum as well, given that Saajan had fucked her in her *batli*,[21] but his semen had not entered her body through there, at that time, but only hours later through her mouth.

We might borrow Jane Guyer's notion of enhancement, which she uses in the context of body decoration in southern Cameroon, to suggest that such fusions offered a certain "lightness of life."[22] Chapter 1 will argue precisely that flirting and fucking outside the confines of domesticity provided succor and sustenance that made life within the domestic bearable. Despite being a formidable institution, the domestic seems a fragile and precarious entity enabled only by a proper expelling of semen. E. Valentine Daniel writes that "one of the causes ascribed to congenital deformities, the birth of weaklings and impotent sons, is the careless expenditure of valuable semen by the father prior to the moment of conception, so that when he joined his wife in order to conceive, he was in short supply of the potent substance."[23]

This rule concerning expenditure is not limited to the householder and his family but applies to the priests as well in E. Valentine Daniel's ethnography. The priest or *acari* who is supposed to consecrate the house must abstain from sexual intercourse because it is a "heating transaction," and violations of such a rule would result in the house being eaten by white ants:

> Sexual indulgence is punished by the destruction of the house by white ants. White ants eat away the beams and woodwork of a house, not only weakening the structure but also leaving behind a leprous appearance. Here, too, the punishment may be seen as befitting the crime. *Karaiyan* ("white ants") is etymologically derived from *karai* ("stain, blemish, defect, impurity, rust"). A piece of wood wasted by white ants has the blemished appearance of a man's skin wasted by leprosy (*kustam*). Furthermore, leprosy is a wasting disease thought to be caused by indiscriminate and promiscuous sexual liaisons, which is exactly what the Acari has been warned against. For in the context of planting the mulaikkal, any sexual relationship, even with one's own wife, is indiscriminate, if not promiscuous.[24]

I cite this as an instance of the "economy of semen," a shorthand that I will use throughout this study to describe the sexual transactions between hijras and their lovers, customers, and young men. Alain Bottéro used the phrase in his study of the semen-loss syndrome of India to highlight the ayurvedic logic that determined the production, retention, and expenditure of this divine nectar.[25] Much has been written about Indian semen—on the dialectic of its retention and consequent potency, proper expulsion for fertility, relation to heat and cold, anxieties about its loss, value, quality—in texts ancient and modern, that a summary would not be helpful, let alone possible, within the limits and concerns of this book.

Lawrence Cohen's essays are exemplary for any work on nonreproductive sexuality in South Asia, and perhaps a more pertinent example of the economy of semen would be the conversation he records in "The History of Semen: Notes on a Culture-Bound Syndrome." A hustler educates Cohen in a park of Benares where men cruise by saying, "These city boys, these sons of great Seths, come with their father's money and I give them something. They take my strength [referring to his semen] and I take some money." Semen in the ethnographic incident becomes an object that finds its equivalence in money when the sexual transactions cut across urban and rural and class divisions. Apart from arguing that the anxieties of semen loss become an orientalist object of imperious public health discourse, Cohen makes an important intervention in creating space for failure in everyday strivings to uphold the model of culture. He relies on Georges Bataille's work to point out that while there are very strong imperatives to retain semen and make it more potent, only its luxurious expenditure allows for life to be lived "against the grain."[26]

The sexual transactions that took place in Bhadrak and Bhawanipatna did not transgress either class or the urban/rural divide, thus we need to take forward Cohen's inspiration by asking how hijras and their lovers accounted for their luxurious expenditure of semen. The "babies" that hijras would refer to in their flirting, the pregnancies they would claim and would refer to in myths, make me invoke rather than engage with the notion of *amogharetas* as an example of the relationship between desire, power, and semen. Wendy Doniger describes this omni-fertile shedding of male seed:

> In Hindu mythology the instances of unilateral female creation are by far outnumbered by unilateral male creation. The male seed is fertile in itself, particularly the seed of a great ascetic who has kept it within him for a long time and is therefore "one whose seed is never shed in vain" (*amogharetas*); that is, he engenders a child every time he sheds his seed, no matter where he sheds it. Even an ordinary man's seed is basically

the source of life, as is evident from the Upanishadic tradition; in Dhar-masastra, too, the seed remains more important than the womb. The seed shed by a powerful male may fall into any of a number of womb substitutes (a pot, the earth, a river or someone's mouth) and produce an embryo.[27]

The idiom of pregnancy that hijras use gives their lovers a sense of being omnipotent, and to the list of places that Doniger recounts where men shed their ever-fertile seed, I would add the rectum as well. This is the picture of sexuality that we must keep in mind, of hijras desiring "bad things," of pro-ducing omnipotent men, when we look at how public health imagined the risk of HIV.[28]

LIVING WITH AND DYING OF HIV/AIDS

Hijras are too often and too easily relegated to positions of marginality as if their lives can be fully contained within the imperatives of survival—with survival being narrowly defined in terms of not dying of AIDS. Hijras re-emerged into prominence in the mid- to late 1990s when the LGBT move-ment of India began appropriating hijras and reframing them as legitimizing historical figures of queerness. The HIV epidemic has reframed hijras not as signifiers of oriental excess but of a sexual excess of a more secular kind. The urgency of the epidemic resulted in hijras being recruited as local ex-perts trained to practice and disseminate safer-sex advice, given that they are associated with selling anal sex. Yet HIV/AIDS did not make itself ap-parent in obvious ways; rather, it formed the background for the moral and ethical dramas that defined the everyday lives of hijras, such as discharg-ing duties of kinship, achieving financial solvency, choreographing love af-fairs, and participating in the sociality of the local world they inhabited. The resulting vulnerabilities posed by contracting HIV was felt in disparate sites, not just at the molecular level, and thus negotiating the grip of the disease on their lives was a social challenge that constantly mutated and reappeared, very much like the virus itself.

When we look at the answers given to the question, "Why do men have sex with men?" in India's National AIDS Control Organization's (NACO) publication titled *Targeted Interventions Under NACP III: Operational Guidelines* for core high-risk groups, the reasons given link Ayurvedic and

Unani understandings of the body such as "pleasure and enjoyment from discharge ('body heat')" to culturally prescribed norms such as, "Wife will not perform anal/oral sex or husband is ashamed to ask." The answers further link the anxieties of pleasure with the substratum economy of semen as it is inherited and understood through the Hindu-Muslim cosmogony, offering reasons such as "anus is tighter than vagina and gives more pleasure," "protecting a girl's virginity, maintaining chastity," and "no commitment to marriage." Other reasons given are "play" and "curiosity."[29] The limit of this economy of semen, to the extent that it does not and cannot offer anything in exchange to hijras, is also the limit of the hermeneutic of desire; thus, it would be more productive to look at this discourse metapragmatically. If we were to ask what hijras receive in exchange for their services, we would in effect be asking what comes after sex; as Lee Edelman reminds us, "'After' thus stands in relation to 'sex' as 'heteronormative' stands to 'queer,' or as 'history' stands to 'repetition,' or the 'social' to the 'antisocial.'"[30]

In Lawrence Cohen's studies of political pornography, the desire to be penetrated cannot find representation where it serves as a metaphor for the realpolitik; in other words, it expresses the position of the Indian Everyman vis-à-vis the political order: metaphorically speaking, he is being fucked.[31] The political pornography addressed by Cohen differentiates oral and anal sex through the exchange of semen and offers a view of the structure and representation of being penetrated:

> Fellatio differs from anal penetration in Holi cartoons. The fellator is represented as actively desiring the submissive position of taking in another man's *ling*, whereas the man who is penetrated is represented as passive and his desire irrelevant. Fellatio sets up an exchange in space— semen for marked abjection—but anal penetration sets up an exchange only in time, and then only if the participants are able under the sign of carnival to circulate and the penetrator to penetrate. Semen, invisible in this genre of representation of anal sex, does not function narratively as a gift.[32]

But this passage is characterizing porn. Through a masterful juxtaposition of ethnographic scenes, Cohen argues that even when the world is divided into the fucked and the fuckers, there are ways to penetrate and be penetrated that are not inscribed with the violence of the world. The present study seeks to explore how the politics of penetration that takes place between hijras and their lovers is lubricated through the invocation of semen that is never shed in vain. Though it is never gifted in the political pornography that Cohen describes, in the social world of hijras, semen does bear fruit in real, mythic, and fantasized time. The sexual transactions between hijras and men, by insisting on the visibility of semen, play out across the axis of time—although inevitably as a failure. Global public health, very much like NACO, fails to imagine why hijras would have sex with men, and why would they fail to use condoms. Apart from the absence of actual material conditions that would make the use of condoms possible, the risk that HIV posed to one's health and future was one of many in the context of poverty.

So much has been written on HIV across disciplines and its risk for hijras, yet public health does not or cannot contain the danger for disease that diffuses and attaches itself to all sorts of objects for the poor. Adam M. Geary's powerful work, which calls for a molecular understanding of HIV, shows that the reason HIV infections among African Americans is staggeringly high is not because of sexual behavior but because of racism. By disaggregating risk from susceptibility and exposure from infection, Geary shows us that HIV is not really about sexuality at all because not everybody having risky sex is susceptible to disease and not everybody who is exposed to HIV gets infected. He writes:

> Poverty and other relations of inequality are literally embodied as ill health and greater susceptibility to infection. The consequences of poverty negatively impact health through multiple avenues, including malnutrition, stress, lack of access to preventive care, lack of care for persistent infections and disease, more environmental poisoning, and greater susceptibility to parasites. These consequences—especially malnutrition and persistent, untreated infections—lend themselves to immunological compromises that leave individuals more susceptible to successful HIV infection if exposed to the virus.[33]

Yet instead of addressing the damages of poverty, psychic or material, at the molecular or macro level, global health continues to implement and fund strategies based on impoverished psychologized understandings of behavioral change and modification. Study after study measures the limited success of these programs at best and complete failure at worst and continues to frame populations at high risk as recalcitrant, to hurl accusations of illiteracy at these poor bodies who now also shoulder the burden of foiling the best-laid plans of experts. HIV is better understood as a watermark throughout this book; even when I am not addressing it specifically, it is always there in the background.[34] For hijras whose lives I describe in these pages, their everyday existence unfolded in the context of poverty, the damages of which were felt at every level, including the molecular level described by Geary.

Hijras portrayed in this book illustrate how sexuality and poverty intersect to make "positive living" a difficult if not impossible goal to achieve. The metaphor of the watermark allows us to see the possibility of contracting and dying of HIV/AIDS as becoming attached to any object or relationship—food not shared by families, infections not treated, medicines not available, condoms tearing, a violent trick, a belligerent policeman at the hot spot, judgmental stares at the ART center, a gossiping HIV counselor. So, even if this might not seem to the reader to be a book on HIV, it is—not only because many of my friends whose lives are depicted here are dead of AIDS, but also because I am describing the precarious conditions of poverty, which can easily take a turn for the worse.

THE FIELD

My fieldwork was conducted among hijras of rural Odisha, one of the poorest states of India, in the district headquarters of Bhadrak and Bhawanipatna. In my first field site, Bhadrak, hijras earned money mainly through selling wares in the vicinity of the shrine of a Muslim saint (*mazar*) and by begging on trains, collecting money on ritual occasions of childbirths and weddings, dancing at religious festivals, and by sex work. Of all the districts in Odisha, Bhadrak has the highest percentage of Muslims, and the several *mazars* that dot its countryside are of particular importance to the lives of hijras.[35] This detail introduces the particular way in which hijras inhabit the Hindu-Muslim universe. Hijras historically have not been easily relegated either through self-identification or through religious practice to either Islam or Hinduism.[36] And while I had both Hindu and Muslim informants, their beliefs and practices would often adhere to one while being claimed as characteristic of the other. Therefore, this book practices a certain fidelity to the way the crossovers between Hindu and Muslim theologies were lived—that is, both as an instantiation and a limit of the notion of religious syncretism. This is changing, as mentioned earlier, as hijras are absorbed into the political agenda of Hindu nationalism.

Let me offer some background to illuminate the mode in which my fieldwork was conducted and to evoke the position of hijras in the social sphere of rural India. My research took place in rural settings where hijras' lives remain immersed within their natal and biological families. The book focuses on sexual economies in rural Odisha and is based on extensive fieldwork conducted between 2008 and 2019. I was able to accompany my informants to different sites their work carried them to, and to participate in the various activities that defined hijra life. We would travel to weddings and childbirth ceremonies across the coastal districts of rural Odisha to sing and dance and collect alms. I was also absorbed in their daily routines of traveling on trains to beg and would spend time with them in the marketplaces and on the highways where they met their clients for sex work.

Hijras in this part of unspectacular India are not expelled by their families because of their sexual lives but rather perform crucial economic functions tied to their sexuality that enable the families' survival. Money they make through begging on trains, at weddings, religious festivals, and childbirth ceremonies and through sex work illuminate an extended erotic economy in which families live through the labor and bodies of hijras. When hijra bodies are considered crucial to sustaining the domestic sphere, we are offered a means of formulating the stakes of nonprocreative sexuality in kinship.

Hijra mobility—because of begging on trains—resulted in my being introduced to other hijras who did not live in Bhadrak but passed through its train station every day. I was able to become friends with one such group of hijras that lived in Jajpur, a neighboring district. My stays in Jajpur were always very brief, primarily because I conducted interviews of hijras of that district while they were resting in Bhadrak, awaiting the train on which they would both beg and return home. Sometimes I accompanied them to Jajpur on the train, then returned in the evening, about a one-hour journey. I also accepted their invitation to stay in the hijra household in Jajpur for two months in 2012, which gave me an opportunity to compare the set of freedoms and restraints that living in a traditional hijra household afforded. Though I met hijras of Jajpur often, I did not stay there as long as I did in Bhadrak and Bhawanipatna. I went to Bhadrak and Jajpur in the summer of 2008, then again in the summer of 2009. During the second trip I went to Bhawanipatna for the first time. I spent sixteen months in these districts from May 2011 to September 2012 and returned for brief visits in the summers of 2013, 2018, and 2019.

I chose to conduct fieldwork in these three districts for several reasons. The first was to study the relationship between hijras and their families. When hijras are initiated into a hijra community or household they are required to sever all ties with their families and natal homes.[37] This separation, however, is overstated, and previous ethnographies—which are discussed at various points in this study—have shown that hijras continue to maintain a relationship with their families in varying degrees and kinds. The second motive was to study how rural settings were becoming more viable than urban locales as a context for hijras to make a living. The figure of the hijra has always been tethered to urban settings, but my research shows that the increasing spread and density of railway connectivity have allowed hijras to make a better living in rural areas than in the cities, where the cost of living is higher and the demands of the traditional hijra communities—in terms of rules to be followed—are more stringent. The third reason was to understand how sexual transactions and affairs were conducted, given the lack of anonymity that marked the rural context. This familiarity with men with whom hijras had sex disturbs the lines of division between categories of lover and customer in several ways. In rural areas there was always the possibility of the customer becoming the lover, and, moreover, the sexual relationship between hijras and their lovers/customers was predicated on other forms of relating—as neighbors, as fellow vendors in the marketplace, or as kin, whether fictive or real.

The constraints of the rural field site explain why the data I have collected takes the form of intimate portraits of a few individuals rather than observations of a large community. Every city in South Asia, large or small, will have its local hijra community comprising groups who share a living space—that is, a household, though not one consisting of biological kin—and in turn will be able to draw their genealogical relationship to the several traditional hijra dynasties of South Asia. The rural setting was a different matter, however. Most of the rural hijras I knew lived with their families. They would, in addition, rent a small room near the train station if their natal homes were an hour or two away. In these rented rooms they would rest between stints of begging on trains and conduct sex work. The second field site of Bhawanipatna, the district headquarters of Kalahandi, did not have a railway station, and here hijras earned their money through sex work conducted in the night along the highway that passed through the district. The numbers of hijras in these three rural districts was small compared to cities but was definitely increasing rather than dwindling.[38]

When I returned to Bhadrak in 2011 for a long stretch of fieldwork, I had great difficulty finding a place to stay. Although I bore all the markings of one not from rural India, my research topic—the sexual lives of hijras— elicited a lot of disapproval. I gave up trying to find a place to stay near the district headquarters, which housed many government officials, and decided to live near my informants in a small settlement called Shankarpur, adjoining the marketplace and shrines of two Muslim saints, Sarkar Baba and Jumman Baba. A certain Mrs. Jain who also lived in Shankarpur and who stitched blouses for a living ran a side business of making bangles. This business was not doing well, and she used to ask Jaina, my primary informant, to read the Koran in the bangle factory and pray for her good fortune. Jaina was given some money every week for this service. Jaina presented me to her as a fellow hijra, and Mrs. Jain offered me a room in the factory in return for my prayers as well. Jaina and the other hijras answered questions about my presence in their company with the reply that I was a hijra as well. This made it easier for me to remain with my informants for long swaths of time while they worked at marketplaces and shrines and to join them when they begged on trains, collected money at shops, and danced at festivals. It was not just my sexuality but also my long hair and female clothing that made me recognizable as a hijra, enabling me to linger amongst hijras next to the highway, where we would have long conversations between their sex work.

MINDING MY LANGUAGE

My fieldwork presented a dilemma with regard to language describing sexuality that is hinted at by Mark Doty in his short story *The Unwriteable*: "I have the language of pornography, I have the language of anatomy or medicine, I have the language of euphemism and I'm happy with none of them."[39] For instance, the English word "sex" was used mostly in the rooms of DAPCU (District AIDS Prevention Control Unit) and other organizations during safer-sex training sessions but not in the public spaces inhabited by hijras. The word *chodhna* was used most often when hijras were talking to hijras, family members, various people in the market, and me in various tones of jest, anger, and seduction. The word "fuck" comes closest to *chodhna* in its pliable polyvalence. The only difference between the uses of the word *chodhna* and "fuck" that I must mention is that while "fuck" in some uses erases the divide of penetrating or being penetrated (as in, "Let's fuck"), *chodhna* would always mean to penetrate. For example, my question posed to hijras, "*Tum kya usko chodh rahi ho?*," which could be translated as, "Are you fucking him?," would result in a lot of giggles because hijras don't or shouldn't and sometimes cannot penetrate but are penetrated. The more accurate conjugation would be "*tum kya use chudhwa rahi ho?*" or "*woh kya tumhe chodh raha hai?*," which would be translated as "Are you getting fucked by him?" or "Is he fucking you?"

Euphemisms were never used by hijras or anybody else, for that matter, to refer to sex between hijras and men, or any illicit sexual transactions. Rather, they were reserved mostly for the relationship between husband and wife. Women would often say to hijras that their husbands were not sleeping with them, not speaking to them, or not coming to them. Hijras, when unsure of how the brazen invitations to fuck would be taken—for example, when they were meeting a man for the first time and wanted to find out whether he would be amenable to fucking—would use the word *kaam*, which would be translated as "work." So, when Shonali struck up a conversation with a young man at a train station by asking the innocuous question, "Are you from Jalasore or are you here for work?," the man answered that his family was in Cuttack but he worked in Jalasore. Shonali then asked in a sweet, coy manner, "*Aapka kaam kaise chalta hai agar bibi se itna dur rehte ho?*," which could be translated literally as, "How does your work get done if you live so far away from your wife?," but a more accurate translation would be, "How do you get by if you live so far away from your wife?" The word *kaam*, therefore, would be used as a metaphor for sex but only in anaphoric speech, in which the metaphoricity was made clear by signaling the "work" that takes place between husband and wife. In other words, *kaam* would be used for "sex" only after the purpose of the conversation had been made clear.

I have used "fuck" rather than "have sex" throughout this book not only to show how rarified the clinical air around intimacy and passion sounded to hijras in their everyday life, but also to highlight that there is a difference between the pleasures of fucking and the pleasures of sex.[40] The endeavor to spread safer-sex information to halt the HIV epidemic has come across difficulties in translating the clinical discourse of safer-sex primarily because the biological is very rarely the universal; scientific-medical discourses about sex have taken different routes as well as different roots across the globe. How, when, and where the clinical has become vernacularized and collo-quialized is thus dependent on differentiating factors such as class, race, caste, and so on.[41] In view of this, I do not want to risk portraying a de-eroticized version of hijras' sexuality because it would confirm rather than dispute the accusations of excess and pathology that have reframed devi-ant sexuality post-HIV. Furthermore, I have tried to show the various ways in which the sexual act was referred to in contexts different from flirting, such as when it became a concern for people other than hijras and their lov-ers, in forms of gossip, rumors, and so on; in such moments sex was re-ferred as "it" or "that."[42]

Despite being one of the most widely recognized features of South Asia at the time of writing this book, hijras have been the focus of anthropologi-cal inquiry in only two book-length ethnographies, by Serena Nanda and Gayatri Reddy, respectively.[43] I redeploy the ethnography from this archive alongside my own to create a conceptual apparatus that shows the sense in which hijras stand in a *diagonal* relation to the symbolic and the social—as instantiated by the family, the state, the married heterosexual couple, and the world at large. I bring themes of erotic-asceticism—which have a long history in South Asian thought—to bear on psychoanalytic and anthropo-logical theory to break through binaries of inside–outside that have long held sway when talking about queer sexuality. Thus, I argue, what is often seen as marginal is actually central and integral to the constitution of the social, and to this extent the book is an invitation to rethink notions of marginality and to broaden the narrow boundaries of reproductive heteronormativity.

By tracking how hijras participate in public spaces, the family, and the state, and in defining the masculinity of their lovers, I show how the bound-aries of the institutions with which hijras interact are permeable, the labor and work of minor actors such as hijras animating these very institutions and giving them life. The theoretical stakes of the book are to reconfigure the manner in which anthropology and studies of South Asia might be aligned to psychoanalytic thinking, although the latter does not remain un-changed in the process. This book is about the small pleasures of everyday life—laughter, flirting, teasing—but also about questions of the queer soul in India, as calls of kinship, duty, and honor draw and quarter it. It interrupts a global discourse with its strong language, which makes hijras commensurable with interventions of HIV prevention, health, and human rights to show that hijra sexuality, though not fully embraced, is nevertheless accommodated by various actors and institutions of the social in terms other than the normal or the pathological.

By studying scenes in the marketplace where flirting between hijras and men of the village takes place, I dispute the readings of marginality ascribed to hijras. Shifting focus from queer son and patriarchal father to the hijra sibling and her brother offers a new way of thinking about the family drama in South Asia. Begging on the trains with them and coinhabiting various other sites where hijras earned their livelihood enabled me to avoid reducing hijra lives to suffocating oppression, and instead to render them in terms of aspirations, for ethical accounting. I spent countless evenings listening to hijras talk about their love affairs—some that failed, some that did not, some that remained unrequited, and some they hoped would eventually become the stuff of legend. I relate these stories to South Asian romances that are part of popular folklore to show that love between hijras and men are not considered out of the ordinary for a large swath of the Indian population obscured by the shorthand the "poor and illiterate."

THE SHAPE OF THE BOOK

Since this book studies the rhythm and flow of everyday life for hijras, its chapters settle on ordinary activities that consume their waking hours. Chapter 1 begins by studying the flirting that takes place between hijras and the men of the village to critique the all-too-easy reading of hijra sociality as an expression of marginalization, exclusion, and stigmatization. I argue that hijras, far from being on the outskirts of society, through their offerings of sexual pedagogy actually reveal to us the dynamics of entering and belonging in the social world—or, in other words, the erotic dynamics between the householder and the ascetic that maps onto the links between the domestic realm and the world outside. The forms of life that hijras inhabit, I argue, in various ways lie both within the larger Hindu and Muslim universe of sociality and outside it—a posture I describe as being diagonal to that world. I then extend the conceptual apparatus of the diagonal in the later chapters in the book. This chapter illuminates the diagonal stance and traces it under a larger ethical rubric of endurance or preservation in several ways. For example, this form of ordinary ethics involves a type of ironic speech that is geared toward producing the aesthetic emotion of *srngara*— or love with laughter as its main foundation (*sthayi bhava*), but one that is subtended with swirling contradictory moods of melancholia, hope, sadness, and euphoria surrounding it.

Chapter 2 studies the relationship that hijras have with various members of their family, focusing on the fraternal bond as it occupies the Archimedean point or pivot that reveals how hijras calibrate their relationship with kin in light of the fact they used to be men, but are not anymore. I argue that the presence of a hijra within the family, gauged through such things as the anxiety of property transmission and inheritance, calls for reconfiguring the accepted notions of kinship, care, and asceticism that often define anthropological investigations of sexuality. I show how anxiety indexes the operations of domestic citizenship because hijras make legitimate claims to ancestral property that must be heeded, but by choosing not to marry and reproduce, hijras opt out of propagating the lineages through which the land is bequeathed. Yet the gesture of hijras' "opting out" of a reproductive future, carried in dominant forms of local kinship, was accompanied by suspicions surrounding their membership in the domestic, as they did sometimes get married, kept or were maintained by wives, and raised children (which their wives had with them or other men) or adopted orphaned children. In this chapter I argue that despite the suspicion and stigma carried in their bodily comportments and practices, hijras participated in transactions that constituted the everyday of households and the domestic sphere. This participation reveals to us the often-hidden emotional labor of building and maintaining familial ties. The sex that hijras have forms a part of nonreproductive affective labor that nevertheless complements and sustains social and familial reproduction.

An interlude maps out how hijras are placed within the male/female binary. It offers a critical examination of the way hijras have been defined— as the third gender, neither man nor woman, and transgender. Here I suggest there are alternative ways of thinking about hijras in terms of other schemas—such as asceticism, eroticism—that lead us away from contradictions arising from identities based on gender and sexuality. My suggestions are based on how claims of being *asli* (real/authentic) or accusations of being *nakli* (false/impostor) are made, depending on context. Being a hijra points to a broader ethical posture, I argue, with resultant impacts on the performance of gender and sexuality. Also addressed here is the way in which hijras frame their sex work and its relation to the formation of their asceticism. I suggest that the boundaries between clients, friends, and lovers tend to become blurred as the intimacy and relationship between hijras and their lovers unfold. This difficulty in clearly separating boyfriends, lovers, husbands, friends, and clients is partly because of the economic relationship between hijras and their world, which is the focus of the next two chapters.

Chapter 3 studies the movement of the money hijras earn and collect that complicates traditional notions of moral-religious exchange such as *daan*, *dakshina*, *bhiksa*, *dalaali*, and *haq*. The intersection of poverty and sexuality embodied in the figure of the hijra has stalled what many would have liked to see become a revolution of social change. The occupations of hijras, through which they earn livelihoods and sustain extended networks of kin, consist of begging and prostitution. Efforts to understand these historically stigmatized positions—the beggar, the prostitute, and the diseased—as pathologies of poverty resulting from discrimination, redressable through legal interventions, have not been taken seriously on the ground by hijras in Odisha. Rightly so, given that not only do these interventions rob hijras of an agential capacity arising out of their sexuality and desire, they also render the goal of the revolution as one that should make hijras bourgeois—a respectable middle-class citizen of the nation-state—thus rehearsing the pedagogical impulses of colonialism in the postcolonial polity. The other figure that emerges, whose rights have not been addressed by the LGBT movement, is the figure of the hijra politician. I read hijras' participation and popularity at the rural-district level, if not at the national level—and the silence that very tellingly surrounds it in the LGBT movement—as reflecting the moral biases invoked in the idea of revolutionary change. The distance created by viewing hijras only as a beggar and not as a politician, I argue, is an invitation to rethink the terrain of morality and ethics as signaled by her discursively split figure. The chapter continues to ask how the figure of the hijra is *enmeshed* in the state—as opposed to simply reiterating her marginality.

Chapter 4 is a study of love affairs and sexual transactions between hijras and their men. I show how it is impossible to draw a boundary around the sexual act in terms of time, space, and experience. By this I mean that the sexual encounter cannot be reduced to penetration, and this impossibility contributes to the failure to use condoms. The social and biological death that an HIV infection implies, in spite of best efforts to destigmatize HIV, is not a sufficient deterrent in the quest of love. This is because the structure of love affairs in South Asia is not just a matter of bodies but also of souls. And because sex and love are also matters for the soul, it participates in several imaginations of time and space that are the basis of religious, mythological, and poetical understandings of love. I show this point by mapping narratives collected from hijras onto medieval Sufi-Hindavi romances like *Madhumalati* and *Mrigyavati*. These romances reveal that the course of love follows a certain design, logic, or sacred geometry that expands love, sex, and attachment to verge on an unbounded experience. By drawing parallels between the love affairs of hijras and Sufi-Hindavi romances, I depict the sexual act between hijras and their partners as something powerful, integral to living and dying, rather than explicating identities through categories such as "high risk" or "MSM." Here I borrow conceptual apparatuses from scholars across disciplines, including literary criticism, queer theory, and anthropology, studying very different contexts to underscore the productivity of desire to argue that if sexuality is differentiated through the striations of class, then we see in the love affairs I describe a reconfiguration of the abjection of poverty.

Chapter 5 revisits the questions regarding HIV raised in the introduction in light of the materials that have been discussed in the chapters. This chapter attends to the form of risk-taking that was inevitable for hijras in available local moral worlds. I juxtapose the risks of living as a hijra with the risk-taking discouraged by public-health authorities in order to measure the distance between the kind of life imagined by the HIV discourse and the one that is lived in rural Odisha. The conclusion presses my ethnographic elaboration and challenge to both public-health discourse and the recent movements in queer theory that focus on temporality and notions of the future. By studying love affairs not only as an instantiation of queer desire but also as an experience of time, I show that the sexual encounter is not so much an act as an event, because its boundaries are never clear. Participation in this event undoes any easy reading, evading the notion of futurity that many queer theorists have positioned at the center of the queer subject. Instead, I argue that love affairs with hijras in some of the poorest districts of India can be seen to transform the experience of time: from a cruel, unforgiving grind directed toward an inevitable abject future to an effervescent present. The overall structure of the book, then, can be seen as follows: the introduction raises the problem of hijra sexuality for HIV prevention as seen through the lens of global public health, the concluding chapter looks at the same issue through the eyes of hijras, and interleaved between these two ways of looking at this topic of critical importance are the chapters that describe everyday hijra lives, struggles, and joys.

1

A PRODIGIOUS BIRTH OF LOVE

This chapter begins by looking at how hijras use laughter, flirtation, and seduction to give an ethical form to their desire for men. Bergson undertakes the task of revealing the logic of laughter—from its inception to its infection—in his *Laughter: An Essay on the Meaning of the Comic* (1900). Laughter, he observes, indicates a slight *revolt* on the surface of social life: "It instantly adopts the changing forms of the disturbance. It also is afroth with a saline base. Like froth, it sparkles. It is gaiety itself. But the philosopher who gathers a handful to taste may find that the substance is scanty and the after-taste bitter."[1] The presence of other people is important for laughter because, as Bergson explains, "our laughter is always the laughter of the group," and if laughter is supposed to be a corrective, since you can laugh at people, then I imagine it would require more than one person. Taking Bergson's cue to study laughter as "a living thing," I show how its slight revolt, corrective, and bitter aftertaste relate to the fucking between hijras and men of Bhadrak, through the following scene:

Each evening many young men who were tired after a long day's work would gather in my room, which was in a local bangle factory, to lounge, chat, and live a bit dangerously by engaging in prurient conversation with Jaina, Azgari, and whoever happened to be visiting. Jaina would inevitably tire of the conversation, a strange mash-up of flirting, sexual proposals, religious diktats, and singing. Jaina would start pretending as if she were in labor, untying her lungi, and, like women do with their petticoats when they go bathing in public, she would tie the lower garment around her neck. She would then start writhing on my straw mat, squealing loudly in cries of pain and grabbing her perfectly round belly. The boys, amused, laughed hysterically and teased her, "Whose child is it, Jaina?," and Jaina would reply either by uttering the name of the boy or coyly gesturing toward him on whom she had harbored a crush for a while (if he was there) or by saying, "The one whose child it is, knows, why don't you go ask him?" (if her current object of lust and affection was not present). Azgari would join, giving advice: "Why aren't you drinking water?—the baby will come out swimming." "Shall I rub soap in your vagina so the baby slips out?" The whole impromptu drama would end with everybody laughing hysterically. I want to consider the implications of this comic performance, the "artificial mechanization" of the body, because, as we shall see, it shores up various other ethnographic instances of conversations and discussions about hijra bodies and the question as to whether she could give birth to children.

Bergson writes that the mechanical and comical emerge from within the contrast of the "irksome ballast" of the body as they meet the "soul eager to rise aloft." The body of the comic illustrates the discomforting disciplines and anatomical limits of the social, which laughter allows us to trespass. The laughter provoked by the pregnant hijra, then, can be read as not just indexing a particular vexed relationship with the world but as enfleshing it in a way that tames the moral impulses carried in kinship. Does depositing semen in the rectum waste its vitality? If so, does the wasteful immorality of hijras fucking—embodying the very obverse of kinship—offer some respite from the morality embedded in kinship? For Bergson, the moral colludes with the social to choreograph bodies, and when they slip out of gear, a dissonance is created that he argues is characteristic of the comic: "Any incident is comic that calls our attention to the physical in a person when it is the moral side that is concerned," and, furthermore, the comic evokes "a person embarrassed by his body." The comic birthing scene in my room can be read as signaling Jaina's disappointment with her body, yet the surrounding men were also the objects of laughter by the amused onlookers (who were always present, since a lot of seduction and flirting happened at the marketplace, usually in Azgari's shop). Not only was the hijra's mechanized body found humorous, but through her statements the body of the youth who refused to indulge in immorality also got laughed at. The laughter is an invitation to men, forwarded by hijras, to enter this cleavage between her body and the social and to enjoy the pleasures of betrayal afforded by the temporary suspension of the moral in this space. The laughter will perhaps allow us to see two things in relationship: first, the force of the moral persuasion of kinship as it simultaneously acts on the body and the social; and second, the tenor and tone of freedoms and constraints that arise through the desire for anal sex (both being penetrated and penetrating) that betrays the moral persuasion of kinship.

I lived behind Azgari's bicycle shop and would often go there to sit and have tea. During these times, she would often start talking loudly about how many boys came to fuck her last night. She would divulge this information in the presence of some boy whose lust she had satiated the night before. Through that satiation and this form of recollection, Azgari was inviting him to come for another visit—one that might be, for her, yet another chance to get the fertilizing fuck that will render her pregnant. When she was trying to seduce someone by provoking him, she might say, "Oh, he used to talk so big about how he would impregnate me at the first shot, fuck me till I wouldn't be able to take it, fuck me so hard that he would send me to the hospital, but when it came the time to do it, his cock was so small"—gesturing with her hand to show the length of her middle finger. The boy at this point, if he had already fucked her, would often start blushing and smiling to himself, concentrating on his bicycle and the task of pumping air into its tires. Usually his friends were near, so they would also tease him: "What did Azgari say? You don't have any power." Size, prowess, virility, and the ability to fertilize were all signified by a large cock. On the other hand, if the boy had not fucked her, she would change the tense of her statements to, "Oh, he talks big but I am sure his is very small, that's why he can't fuck me, that's why he doesn't come—how will he come, sister [turning to me], what will he do if he comes?—he is so small he can't fuck." The reaction of the boys would usually be the same as toward their counterpart who *had* fucked her. The laughter in this case was directed toward those who stubbornly refused to become men by refusing the rite of passage of losing their virginity to one of these old bawdy pushy hijras. Usually the poor youth was forced by the merciless teasing of friends to prove Azgari's claims wrong by—as luck would have it—fucking Azgari herself. This is how Azgari and the laughter she provoked would, in Bergsonian terms, "correct men's manners."

The correction tendered by Azgari, which can be seen as repositioning her lovers from following one set of rules to another, operates in the mode of seduction. Seduction cajoles one into committing acts that are not definitively marked by either coercion or consent. I offer the following ethnographic incident, which I want to study in terms of the corrective qualities of a hijra's seductive wiles. Once, soon after I had reached Bhadrak in 2011, Shamsheri asked me to take her to buy some slippers, and I agreed. At the shop, a charming young chap not much older than fifteen, but with the airs and efficiency of a much older person, was helping her while the shop owner was sitting and chatting with a friend of his. Shamsheri started flirting with the boy by accusing him of showing her substandard slippers, which the chap denied, to which she then said, "You make everything I say into lies." The young man smiled, puzzled, and asked to which statements she was referring. Shamsheri replied, "You refused to acknowledge the unborn child in my stomach as yours, you say I am lying when I tell you it's yours." The owner and his friend, who were talking nearby, started laughing as the boy blushed with embarrassment. This encouraged Shamsheri, and she continued, "Do you deny you come to my house at night?" The owner asked, "Really?" Shamsheri replied, "Yes, of course, ask him. In the middle of the night he will keep on knocking on my door, waking everybody up and dragging me to the field; he won't let go of me till the morning breaks." The owner and his friend started laughing and teasingly caught the boy by the scruff as the boy turned to Shamsheri, asking with a laugh, "Why are you dragging my name through mud?" Shamsheri, as a parting shot, threatened that she will throw the baby in the river; when people ask her about it, she will put all the blame on the boy because he refused to acknowledge his paternity, and she was rendered helpless.[2]

I found the boy's response interesting, since he did not outright deny the accusations leveled against him; instead, his reply was, "Why are you dragging my name through mud?," which could be seen as a mild reprimand against Shamsheri for making public the secret of their sexual affair—secrecy that Alfred Gell has suggested is central to any love affair.[3] If the accusations are false, then through her playful teasing, ostensibly made to generate laughter, Shamsheri had made known to the boy that she was interested in having sex with him. The boy in turn, by not denying the accusation, made it known that both were possibilities—and the night to come suddenly seemed full of promise. This ambiguity in the boy's response and the (im)possibilities that emerged from it allow the incident to be framed as flirting, consistent with the sense that Georg Simmel lays out:

> The distinctiveness of the flirt lies in the fact that she awakens delight and desire by means of a unique anti-thesis and synthesis: through the alternation or simultaneity of accommodation and denial; by a symbolic, allusive assent and dissent, acting "as if from a remote distance"; or, platonically expressed, through placing having and not-having in a state of polar tension even as she seems to make them felt concurrently. In the behavior of the flirt, the man feels the proximity and interpenetration of the ability and the inability to acquire something. This is the essence of "price." With that twist that turns value into the epigone of price, flirtation makes this acquisition seem valuable and desirable.[4]

The boy's reply reveals his positioning in the world, which is susceptible to change. Shamsheri's words don't fall on deaf ears; they are absorbed, and through that absorption the boy reveals that the terms in which he sees the world can shift or be corrected. What was previously not there—the figure of the hijra in the landscape of pleasure—has now through flirting made an appearance.

A certain agony attends the moment when one's picture of the world is shifted through this correction, enabled by seduction. Margaret Trawick, for example, alludes to the agonizing quality of seduction and love when she writes of her teacher and informant, Themozhiyar:

> Themozhiyar saw himself as my guru and me as his student. He wanted me to believe in his god and to follow his path toward that god. . . . When I was still in Madras, he had performed initiation (*gurudiksha*) on me, by surprise and against my mild protests, by giving me a secret mantra of twenty syllables. I accepted the role of disciple, as being the most appropriate one under the circumstances, though as I got to know Themozhiyar better I found it increasingly difficult to bow to him, even as a nominal gesture. I argued with him frequently, as did his other students, but I was probably more vehement and stubborn than they. I wanted to learn from him, but I also wanted to be in control of the situation in which the two of us found ourselves. I told him that he should consider

me a child, that in my ignorance of Tamil culture I *was* a child, and needed to be taught everything from the foundation up. Themozhiyar agreed to that. I acted as humbly and innocently as was possible for me. But I did not enjoy being treated as an inferior.[5]

Further on, she notes, "The poem [the secret mantra] is also about the love between guru and disciple, how each travels a long way and changes very much in order to meet the other, how each out of love, causes pain to the other, how each, out of love, endures this pain" (23).

In this drama of seduction, a certain agony can be detected that lends itself to be read as sexual pedagogy that shifts somebody's picture and protocols of the world. The following is an ethnographic example that I want to examine as one instance of sexual pedagogy between a hijra and lover. Jaina would say:

A hijra can never set up a house with a man. He is a man, he requires children, heirs, he requires *din-duniya* (religions/customs and world/society). With a hijra, he will not have any children, he will not be able to set up his *duniya* (home/world) with her. But then, not all men are the same; very rarely, there is one in a million who forsakes *din-duniya* and the desire to have children and sets up a house with a *maichiya* and marries her.[6] But then they can't desire anything else, they don't think about anything and can spend their days in the manner they want. Every man, no matter how much he loves a hijra, and no matter how long they live as husband and wife, must leave her to set up *din-duniya*. Look at my case, I spent ten years with Kutty—as husband and wife we lived. He wouldn't eat anywhere but from my hand. The whole world knew. But his sister's husband came to me once when he had gone to Balasore and said, "Look, Jaina, Allah and I know how pure your love is but Kutty will need to set up his home, settle down according to religion/law/customs of the world; he will need to worry about children. If you won't help us in convincing him to get married, he will never get married." In the night, his sister and mother came to me, pleading me to convince him to get married. He was always refusing to get married. So I told him, "I will live with you, I will do *this* whenever you want, wherever you want, but settle down, you will have children, you need to work for your future, what will you get staying with me, I can't give you children or heirs, this is wrong, what is all this?" He said, "You want me to get married, you go find a woman." So, when the marriage was happening, I went to the place with the family, and when they asked, "Who gives the permission for this marriage?" they pointed toward me. I was so embarrassed because it is the mother's or the father's right to give permission. But Kutty said, "No, Jaina will have to give the permission." So I got them married and came back. After the marriage celebrations Kutty, that bastard, landed up at my place in the middle of the night and refused to go to his wife. I was scared for the girl's side, since they were staying with Kutty's family.

They, the brothers of the girl, came to look for him; they told me, "Please send him home, it's one in the morning," but he wouldn't leave. I was in such a fix, what if they get angry, it takes only a second for men to become animals, what if they kill me for stealing their son, brother, brother-in-law? I was so scared that they would become abusive and wake up the entire village. Won't it cause trouble if he doesn't go to his wife? He has gotten married, people will abuse him if he doesn't go to his wife. So, I figured out how to send him; I started touching his penis, pleading all the while—when he got hot, I quickly had sex with him—then I told him to go to his wife. He went away. God knows what he did with her, he was back at my place with the morning *azaan*. I thought, this guy is going to get me beaten up, bastard. I told him, "At least spend the first night completely with your new wife." He said, "shut up," and slipped into my bed. Men will always go to women, there is nothing to feel sad about in this. This is the world's *dastoor* (ways/tradition/rule) and we are *barkhi-laaf* (out-of-joint/out-of-step/against) in this *dastoor*. What to do? *Allah pak* has made us *maichiyas*, but to marry men is not our work, *this* is our *shauq* (enjoyment), marrying men is not what *Allah* made us able to do, it is very wrong; for men to set up *din-duniya* is not wrong.

This story illustrates the agonizing quality of seduction and the antagonism inherent in the flirting: Along with the invitation to participate in a carnality that frees the body from the disciplines of the moral and the social, hijras must remind the boy of the constraints and the risks he runs in renouncing the moral altogether. Hijras must calibrate the relationship in such a way as to push the young lad back into the world, so that he can become the householder, if he is not one already. Calibration refers to the etiquette through which risks and freedoms can be negotiated to sustain not only the social, but also the carnal that refuses to stick amicably to the social. The calibration of etiquette allows carnality that might possibly fracture the social to be absorbed while retaining its odd quality. An instance of calibration or etiquette can be seen in Malinowski's *Sex and Repression in Savage Society*, in which he mentions a variety of sexual taboos in the Trobriands and the varying charges of moral shame attached to them. While the incest between brother and sister threatens the futurity of the social, Malinowski is still able to document an incident in which the siblings "were able to brave it out and lived in incest for several months till she [the sister] married and left the village."[7]

He could not document any incidents of mother-son incest, but there were many instances of breaking the exogamous rules called *suvasova*, which resulted in shame and "eruption of boils all over the body." Thankfully, there was magic to cure the bodily affliction, and the shame for the woman was accompanied with admiration for the man's plucky nature. The case of the infraction of the incest taboo was resolved through the sister's marriage. The sexual act within the household must be carefully positioned within axes of kinship and generational distance to resist incest and result in a viable child, family, and future, because incest can be calculated very widely through rules of *gotra* exogamy in India. The sexual act outside the house, between a hijra and her lover in a space that is literally a field adjoined to the house or the neighborhood and that I call the fucking fields, must also be calibrated, albeit in a different way. If not, then sex with hijras in the fields threatens men with a formless future—a protracted social death. The men won't desire anything else; they won't have any responsibilities or worries and will spend their days in the manner they want. The etiquette to avoid incest and sodomy points to a contradiction at the heart of the social—and the revelation of this contradiction is the pedagogic lesson common to both the myth of incestuous sex studied by Malinowski and the narrative of sex with hijras.

In the primal myth of death-dealing incest, according to Malinowski, the incest between sister and brother results in making two spots on the island sacred: one has two springs and the other contains a ritually important plant that grows from the chest of the dead sibling-lovers. Lovers who want to make sure that their love will be successful or reciprocated must bathe in the spring and conduct a ritual using the leaves of the plant. The incestuous sex and the subsequent death of the siblings make the land fertile and sacred, or, in other words, make life possible for future lovers. The rule of incest is broken, and the incestuous siblings die, but what kills them makes life possible for another future lover. Incest also determines the social etiquette of siblings in the Trobriands: brother and sister are supposed to avoid inquiring about and addressing each other directly—to ward off the threat or suspicion of incest—even though they are inextricably linked with each other for life. This contradiction arising from the incest and sodomy taboos—in which death of incestuous and hijra lovers, in the following myths, results in life for others—is one around which the social congeals and gains its kinetic force by elaborating sets of rules to avoid those two taboos. What is this form of etiquette accomplishing? Is this the force of the moral that anthropologists have articulated in kinship? What are the threats that emerge from the social that endanger it, and how do hijras domesticate them? Let us begin by studying the etiquette, the threats to the social that it wards off, the contradictions that etiquette both hides and reveals, and the resolutions that are offered in the fucking fields where hijras meet their lovers.

The following sections will read the myths that hijras recite as an allegory of what kinds of love survive and the ones that must necessarily die.

THE DEAD BABIES

Every evening, in multiple ordinary conversations that would take place, hijras would refer to their baby all of a sudden, much to the amusement and giggles of everyone present, and this would often be the flirtatious reminder to everyone, in case they had forgotten, that they were invited to impregnate her, or at least fuck her, knowing that one possibility was pregnancy. Sometimes in the late evenings Jaina, if in an exceptionally licentious mood, would stand in the middle of the road and lament loudly, "*Aao re—seat khali hai—baccha kar do*" (Come on—there is an empty seat/vacancy—impregnate me). The following are some of the examples of how the baby was mentioned by hijras:

(a) When Shamsheri refused tea offered by Azgari, she said, "No, the baby will get burnt" (*Nahin baccha jal jayega*), referring to the *tamsik* or heat-producing quality of tea.
(b) When a handsome boy came, wanting to buy flowers, Jaina said, "Come, impregnate me" (*Aao Baccha kar do*), signaling how enamored she

was with him, but also mildly irritated by the fact that he was businesslike with her and would not respond to her flirtations.

(c) When someone asked Azgari how she was, she answered, "The baby dried up" (*Baccha sukha gaya*).

(d) When I asked her whether she was a bit mad (crazy), Jaina referred to herself in the third person, saying, "Somebody has abandoned Jaina after getting her pregnant" (*Jaina ko koi pet se kar ke bhaag gaya*).

(e) When Jaina asked me, "What are you writing?" Akhtari replied, "She is making a baby/fucking" (*Baccha karti hai*).

(f) Once Mangu, who lives in Charampa, was dropping me off at the auto stand so that I could go back to my hut. She started flirting with an incredibly handsome young auto-rickshaw driver. The man giggled amusedly and playfully pretended to punch Mangu's stomach. She squealed, "What if the baby gets hurt?" (*Baccha ko lag jayega toh?*)

(g) Jaina wanted to send a message through a mutual friend to a boy, Akbar. When the friend asks why the boy should come to meet Jaina, she screams, "He has left me pregnant, now he won't even come to take care of me" (*Baccha kar ke chor diya abhi khayal kaun karega?*). When the boy comes, she says, "You have left your baby in my stomach, won't you take care of me: bring me some fruits, bananas, pomegranates, milk, butter, meat?" The boy, irritated by this rubbish, leaves, and Jaina is left amused and a bit embarrassed by this careless and unnecessary insult.

Statements about "the baby," references to the pregnant state of hijras, did not surprise any of us who were lolling about because they happened every day and would be an established pathway of humorous disruption of mundane daily concerns. Disruptive because even when it was not unintelligible, it would appear all of a sudden; and even if it wouldn't surprise us, it would make us laugh. Bergson, in his analysis, wrote, "In a comic repetition of words we generally find two terms: A repressed feeling that goes off like a spring and an idea that delights in repressing the feeling anew."[8] Might we read the frequent reappearance of this ghostly baby as a form of repetition? And if so, then might we read the flirting and fucking as sustaining for the social body, in Lévi-Straussian terms, the animal in the human to be repressed and released? Or, in other words, the baby and in turn the future it promises attenuate the bestial hijra, suturing it to the social but never squaring with it.

The way that Jaina, Shamsheri, and I would amuse ourselves in the hot summer months would be by playing tricks on a certain blind old *maulvi* (religious scholar). Whenever we came across him in our before-lunch rambles in the early afternoon, Jaina would drag me in front of him and say, "Oh *maulvi saheb*, please breathe on her, she is not managing to get pregnant." The *maulvi saheb* would touch my head with my long hair bunched up and would be convinced that I am a woman and would breathe and mumble some lines, while Jaina and Shamsheri were at pains to control their laughter. Eventually they would burst out laughing hysterically, while I would look amused at this trick, which was growing old after the twentieth time we had done it. Jaina would utter breathlessly, "Oh, you're sure to get pregnant tonight." In the marketplace, "the baby" was in many instances invoked as an invitation to flirt, to flatter men about their virility, or to provoke them into proving their prowess, but as I have mentioned, it was also pedagogic.

The trick that Jaina and Shamsheri played on the blind *maulvi* was perhaps an instance of turning the world upside down, a way of negotiating the chafing of the social. The bestial hijra reminds her lover that the world, the family, and the household are all a game, but a game that he must necessarily play. As Lee Siegel writes:

> There is always a trickster in the game, a joker in the deck to prevent the rules from becoming oppression, the contest from becoming tedious or dull in losing its surprises and enchantments. . . . Through his lies, pranks, games, and jokes, turning the world upside down, the trickster— divine, human, or bestial—in the heavens, court, market, village, or jungle—is the guardian of humor, prompting us to laugh at ourselves, to take nothing seriously, to realize that profundities are but vain inventions of desperate intelligence. He exists in order to remind us of the game, that the game is all.[9]

Hijras were somewhat like tricksters whose flirting and pranking made a joke of rules and norms and thereby relaxed one's grip on everyday life and made living possible. Hijras' fucking is a constant reminder that the rules of the game are never in one's favor; the carnal, even though mediated through the social, will never sit with it comfortably. The stakes, hijras remind their men, are mortal, and they entail enduring a social that at its heart exacts a cost that cannot be survived intact.

Whenever I would tie my laundry into a small bundle, Jaina would insist on taking it to the launderer. Her insistence, I later found out, stemmed from the fact that there were various men in that neighborhood with whom she would spend hours flirting and whiling away the evening. I discovered her flirtations after thinking it odd that she considered my clothes *napaak* (unclean)—meaning she would never touch my clothes, insisting that I tie the bundle—yet she had no problem with carrying it, refusing my offer to drop it off myself. Whenever she would pick up the bundle she would start reciting the same old lines in the same manner of loud lamentation: "Oh, why are you asking what's in the bundle? My baby is in the bundle, I suffered a miscarriage last night." If she was not in a hurry and there was an audience, the recitation would become an extempore: "My husband beat me up so brutally because I miscarried the baby—I am taking the bundle to the river to throw it away—what else can I do?"

As usual, this bit of drama would cause a lot of laughter and could last from five minutes to an hour, depending on the size of the audience and the amount of encouragement their laughter provided. But the reference to the dead fetus took another tone when Jaina recounted this incident from her past to me:

When I was very young, I hadn't gotten into this sort of *work* then. I was very young, must have been thirteen or fourteen. I was very beautiful and Siddhiqui had called me home. When I went there, I saw these two handsome men; I knew them, but they were rich, I was poor. I used to work at that time in Kaalu's hotel. Remember I had taken you there? Yes, Kaalu's father used to run it. I didn't know but Siddhiqui had called me because the men wanted to get "work" done [*kaam karwana chahte the*, meaning that the men wanted to have sex; *kaam*, "work," was the metaphor most often used to denote sex]. I had not experienced any sex then, I was just told that Siddhiqui wanted to see me. When I arrived, there was lots of good food, alcohol, paan, and so on. They all spoke very nicely to me, then Siddhiqui went outside, the men started touching me and kissing me and I liked it very much. There was also desire in my mind. They were also young, then they grabbed my breasts and I didn't know what was happening, my body was on fire, but when they pushed it inside, I couldn't take it, I tried to tell them to stop but they had their hands on my mouth. After they were both done, I was in a lot of pain and I was crying and there was blood everywhere. Siddhiqui heard me cry and came inside and screamed at the men, "He is a child, you should have been gentle, it was his first time, how could he have taken it so quickly? You should have put it inside slowly. Is this any way to treat somebody when they are not used to this sort of work?" The men felt very bad and gave me some money and left. Siddhiqui asked me to sleep over because if I were to go home there would have been questions about the blood on my clothes and why I had been crying. So, I slept there. Siddhiqui himself washed my clothes that night and left them to dry. Soon, I became unwell, my head was spinning, I was vomiting, everything I ate would come out. My stomach was aching all the time, medicine was not helping. I didn't know what was happening. After two or three months, I went to shit in the field and I was in so much pain that I fainted. The other people I worked with came looking for me, including the hotel's owner, Kaalu's father. The next morning, he called me and asked me what had I been up to. I replied nothing and he said that I should tell him truthfully, otherwise he will beat me. I was young, so I told him what had happened. He then went in search of those two men and when they came, he shouted a lot at them, and told them that when he picked me from the field, he saw that an embryo had come out of my body. You won't believe what a *karishma* (miracle) had happened, Vaibhav, it was an embryo. They were shocked and said that was impossible, so he took them to the field, and showed them. They were young, they didn't know what *bacche ka chala* (an ulcer of pregnancy) looks like. They said the old man was just making it all up, so the old man asked whether he should call other people and ask them to tell them what it was? They got scared and requested that he forgive them. He gave them a warning and let them go.

The most poignant story I heard about a hijra's pregnancy came from Lovely Kinnar. Lovely was considered by far the most beautiful hijra in the six districts of coastal Odisha connected by the Calcutta–Madras train route. Word about her beauty had spread far and wide, and Lovely was well aware of it. She was always beautifully dressed in shimmering saris; the birth-control pills that hijras take had a very good effect on her face, which was without any facial hair and was not at all pockmarked by the constant *darsan*.[10] The breasts that she grew were a nice commendable size; they would have only grown bigger if she had done silicone. We all looked at her with much envy. I would always stay with her when I went to Jajpur; her room had one bedroom and a kitchen. The walls of the bedroom were very pink, and one of them was covered with a large plastic poster of a white naked baby with blue eyes. It had always been there, but I had never inquired about it until now, provoked by all the babies bandied about in conversation. I turned to her and asked, "Why do you have this poster?" Lovely flicked her doll-like eyes up from cutting vegetables and said:

> Last year, I had great pain in my stomach, no medicine would help, everybody thought I was pregnant; Guruma thought I was pregnant as well because the symptoms were exactly that of pregnancy, you know, like the ones pregnant women have. I was vomiting, my head was spinning, I couldn't eat, everything I would eat would be vomited.[11] Guruma even conducted a puja to our goddess thanking her for the miracle in allowing this pregnancy to happen. My husband and I, upon the Guruma's advice, bought this poster because if you look at a beautiful baby when you're pregnant then your baby will also be beautiful. My husband took me to the doctor and because I look like a lady, after I told the nurses the symptoms they all told me I was most probably pregnant and the doctor asked me to wait so that he could see inside with the computer. I did not tell them that I was a hijra. When the doctor was looking inside my stomach, and in the computer, he looked very confused because he could see that there was no child. He said to the nurses, "Lovely Sahoo is a man." The nurses looked at him and said, "But this is Lovely Sahoo." "I know," the doctor said, "but Lovely Sahoo is a man." They didn't know I knew English, both the nurses looked at me astonished and did not know what to say. They kept on staring, and the doctor then gave me some medicine, and Aijaz and I returned. When we came back, everybody was very sad, but they also made fun of me. Guruma said, "This is what Jagannatha wanted." But I was very sad, you know, for a moment I believed as well that I was pregnant. I know it is impossible but for a few days I had hoped that it was true, what everybody was saying, that I was pregnant. I never got rid of the poster. She went to the poster and said, "Now this is our baby," she pinched the poster baby's penis and said triumphantly,

"When you grow up, tear everybody's cunt." She whipped around and went to cook.

Hijras' babies did not always cause amusement and humor. When one's audience is not the young men with whom one is flirting or in love, or when the scene is not that of seduction, then the story often turns wistful, as Lovely's did; she almost believed that she had been pregnant. Akhtari told me this story on a hot afternoon when she was uncharacteristically despondent.

At Chishti's shrine in Ajmer [i.e., the shrine of Khwaja Garib Nawaz][12] there lives a *sadaa suhaagan* [one who is married/not a widow]; she is a hijra. She is not actually married to a man or the baba, but she dresses that way; her wrists are full of bangles and her body covered in beautiful gold jewelry. A person has to go and plead to her and say, "*Suhaagan*, we don't have a child; please ask the *khwaja* [spiritual master] to bless us with a girl or boy, whichever they want." If somebody wants a child they have to go to the *dargah*, the *khazim* [caretaker] over there will direct them to the *suhaagan*. Then the *suhaagan* will start pleading to Allah: "O Allah, look, this woman has come, asking for a child; it's been so long since she married, why haven't you given her a child?" She will become very passionate in her pleadings. She is very beautiful, more beautiful than women. She will not leave till it becomes Allah's wish to give the woman a child. She will remove her jewelry and break her bangles in *josh* [zeal/passion] asking Allah, "tell me are you going to give a child or not?" Finally, Allah will change his mind and say, "Go, girl, go home, in nine months you will have a child in your lap." After Ramzan, during Eid, the first shroud at the *khwaja saheb* has to come from a hijra, a *maichiya*, otherwise the stove will not catch fire; nobody will be able to make the wood burn for the feast. Nobody else is supposed to put the first shroud besides a hijra.

There was a *maichiya* that used to live with Chishti [Khwaja Garib Nawaz]; she was well versed in the Qur'an, so her name was Hafiz Jamal, but she was a hijra. She had started talking to a rich man's son, and soon they became lovers. Both of them were very beautiful. Soon, people got to know that they were in love, the villagers went to the *seth* [businessman], "Your boy is roaming around with a hijra, aren't you scared he will become spoilt?" The man went to his son and asked why he was roaming around with a hijra. The son replied, because he loved her, why are you displeased with this? "No, people are starting to talk, you are my son and she is a hijra, she is not a woman, what can she give you" [*Tumhara usse kya kuch hoga*]. The son replied, but she is also beloved by *khwaja saheb*, like all of us. The boy and the hijra both went to the *khwaja* and told him, "This is a *seth*'s son and I am a hijra. You know everything about me. Do one thing, give me a child of my lover in my stomach, that looks exactly like my lover, and as soon as I give birth, kill me."[13] After a few days, she was pregnant. They went to the doctor who was very surprised. He took the baby out through an operation. After the child was born, the word had to be kept that she had to die, but as she has asked, the world knew that a hijra had given birth to a child. The child died as well along with the mother. But the whole world knew that her love was true because *khwaja saheb* had given her a child. Her *mazar* [tomb] is still there and it is written, Hafiz Jamal Bibi, now that she had become a mother.

Me: "What happened to the boy?"
Akhtari: [*looking a bit confused*] "He got married to someone else."
[*Here I was a bit surprised and extremely disappointed that he hadn't killed himself because of the pain of being separated from his beloved, but Akhtari didn't register that and was lost in her story.*]
Akhtari: "Since then hijras' *chaddhar* is the first *chaddhar* to go on the shrine on the tenth day of Rajab, three months after Muharram."

There are many different versions of this story floating around. The other version, recounted by Gayatri Reddy in her ethnography conducted in 1995, goes as follows: "There was once a hijra named Tarabai who desperately wanted children of her own. So she went to Ajmer Baba and asked for this wish to be granted. Only, she said, 'I want a child to be produced in my womb,' and did not explicitly ask for it to be born. So her pregnancy continued for several months and finally, unable to bear the pain and burden any longer, Tarabai slit her stomach and removed the baby, killing herself and the baby. But to this day, hijras who go to Ajmer Baba's *dargah* inevitably pay homage to Tarabai as well."[14] Yet another version was told to Serena Nanda when she was conducting her ethnography in 1981:

In Ajmer, in North India, there is a holy place that belongs to hijras. It is called Baba Darga, and it is on top of a hill. One time, during Urs, many people were going up the hill to pay respects to Baba. One hijra was also there. She saw a lady with four children and offered to carry one or two of them. The lady became very angry and told the hijra, "You are a hijra, so don't touch my children." This made the hijra feel very sad, so she asked Baba for his blessings for a child of her own. But she only asked for a child and didn't ask Baba to bring the child out. The pregnancy went on for ten months, and her stomach became very bloated. She went to the doctors but they didn't want to perform an operation [Caesarean section] on her. Eventually she couldn't stand the weight any longer so she prayed to the Baba to redeem her from this situation. But Baba could only grant her the boon, he could not reverse it. When the hijra felt she could stand it no more, she found a sword at the darga and slit herself open. She removed the child and placed it on the ground. The child died and the hijra also died. Now at this darga prayers are performed to this hijra and the child and then to the Baba.[15]

There is yet another widely circulated version, but one that you will never hear from hijras. The *khwaja saheb* was mocked by a hijra that he was no saint and he could perform no miracles, challenging him that if he could perform miracles, then he should be able to make her pregnant. The hijra got pregnant, but because she could not give birth since she had no vagina, she prayed to *khwaja* to relieve her and asked for his forgiveness. The *khwaja* could not take the child back, so she died along with the baby inside her. But since then, hijras have flocked every year to pray and ask for the *khwaja's* blessing.

The Chishti *dargah* is not the only one associated with myths or legends of saints, and their ability bestows fertility on hijras. I was told a similar story of the saint Ganj Rawan Ganj Baksh, whose shrine is near Aurangabad. His powers to bestow fertility were mocked by a hijra as well, who then found herself to be pregnant and, as the story goes, gave birth—but both she and the baby died in childbirth. As in Ajmer, the tombs of the hijra and the baby are near the shrine, and the fruits of the trees of this shrine are supposed to make an infertile woman pregnant. Similar to the workings of the primal myth of incest in Malinowski, which becomes the basis of socially sanctified love—the one that renews the social—the dead hijra and her baby offer a resolution when the social threatens death in the form of infertility—a resolution riddled with pathos because it is also an allegory of what is survivable.

Each version, differing ever so slightly, was told to make a point to the anthropologist. For Malinowski, the slight variations point to a complete cultural formulation, or "picture"; for example, Reddy's informants told her the story to make comprehensible to her that hijras were different from women. Reddy analyzes the story to ask, "Are hijras primary agents of gender subversion in the Indian cultural context, or are they uncritically reinscribing gendered categories through their desires and practices?" She concludes that hijras' "gender performances instantiate their 'inherently ambiguous' and axial position in the Indian imaginary."[16] While a great deal of scholarship reiterates the point about the "ambiguous nature" of hijras, and some do it with good intentions, these formulations end up reproducing categories of resistance and subversion and resignification of the "already given" to forefront the normative in Indian sexualities. But suppose we make a different move instead and locate hijras within the larger Indian imaginary, asking how in Akhtari's story religious idioms and myth make comprehensible the topography of desiring men, revealing pathos in such desires that can never achieve currency. In Simmel's words, desires that cannot twist themselves into a price and hence acquirement, exchange, and possession can only lead the desiring subject to her death—as shown in the stories earlier—but deaths from which the social sustains itself and ensures fertility and futurity.

While Reddy's analysis is precise and helps us to realize that hijras have placed themselves outside the complementarity of the male–female, we will need to place it next to Nanda's conclusion that focuses instead on the register of asceticism of hijras. Doing so, hijras appear not only outside the male–female binary, but also outside the project of the family and its various economies and moral constraints. Nanda writes of the story, "On the one hand it [the myth] expresses the wish of some hijras to have a child, yet, on the other hand, acknowledges its impossibility. The death of the hijra and her child suggests that hijras cannot become women—in the most incontestable sense of being able to bear a child."[17] But one may nonetheless ask, how can one respond to impossible desires and longings? The impossibility of a desire that does not cool no matter how discouraging the evidence and tugs at the carnal to seek comfort, solace, release—making a claim of a different sort on the subject and on the anthropologist.

There are two sets of concerns that I want to study here, the first being the contiguity between the god, the *khwaja*, the hijra or the *sadaa suhaagan*, and the couple that want a child. The asceticism of the *khwaja* and the asceticism of the hijra in Ajmer come together to bestow the infertile couple with a baby; fruits growing from trees near the grave of the pregnant hijra in the *mazar* of Aurangabad grant fertility to an infertile woman. Lives and families are lived in the wake of dead hijras and their babies; the wood in familial hearths will continue to burn only when hijras have given their shroud to the *khwaja*. The form of the hijra's exhortations to the *khwaja* are telling; they can also be read as flirtatious, sweetly coercing the god to bless the infertile couple with a child. The *khwaja* is similar to the hijra to the extent that his desires are focused toward God; as a consequence of this, he steps out of the domestic and participates in a different set of kin obligations than that of husband to wife, father to children, and so on. In the story Akhtari told me, the miracle-giving powers of the *khwaja* are relied on to bring meaning to the claims of love that a hijra feels toward her man. The father interrupts the love affair by saying that the hijra will not be able to give anything or will be useless in the task of setting up a home. He dismisses the love precisely because it cannot transform the man into a father or a householder and thus push him into the economy. The hijra then has to make visible her love, and it is this act of making visible that also gives value to her love in a form that will be recognizable by the father—who is here standing for the social. She does so by giving birth to a baby. But the baby and the hijra *both* must necessarily die, because the point of the child was to show the world that the love was true, that the love was valuable. The implication of this death is that perhaps the love between hijras and their lovers cannot survive in the realm of visibility and value; it can only endure in the darkness of night. It can only exist in invisibility and outside economy, exchange, and value—like the one in a million men that Jaina spoke about, who falls in love with a hijra and leaves the world of men to spend his remaining life doing whatever he wants.

In the last version of the myth that features a hijra mocking the saint, the hijra becomes the skeptic: she questions the value of the *khwaja*'s grace and his proximity to God. The *khwaja* is then called upon to give visibility/value to his love for God. He does so through a miracle; he makes the hijra pregnant, but once again this sign of love—the hijra's baby—cannot survive in the realm of visibility/value, nor can it gain entry into the public or a foothold in the social, hence both the witness and the visible form of that love must die. The *khwaja* and the hijra are, then, not only contiguous but congruent as well in the way their desires find a moment of visibility, but then quickly disintegrate to return to a priceless world, which is free of questions of value and fruition. It is the inextricability of value and the baby that prevents a hijra's love from having any currency.[18] In other words, her love will never become valuable because she cannot have babies, and the moment she does, she will not remain a hijra anymore, she will become a woman—a possibility impossible to sustain even with the help of God. This set of myths also offers us a key to understanding the love between hijras and their lovers. If the *khwaja* and his god are placed exactly in the same position as the hijra and her lover, then we might ask what the implications are that same-sex desire and love carry in this site where the lover is deified.

The *sadaa suhaagan* is the point where the *khwaja* and hijra meet; this figure reveals the form of loving that Akhtari's myth was signaling. The following are a few lines from the poetry of the Sufi Madho Lal Husain to illustrate the figure of the *sadaa suhaagan*:

> *Shak gia beshaki hoi ta mai augan nacci na*
> *je shahu nal mai jhumar pava sada suhagan sacci hai*
> *jhuthe da mukh kala hoya ashak di gall sacci hai*
> *shak gia beshaki hoi ta mai augan naaci hai.*[19]

> The doubt has vanished and doubtlessness is established, therefore I, devoid of qualities, dance.
> If I play (thus) with the Beloved I am ever a happy woman [*sadaa suhaagan*].
> The liar's face (he who accuses) has been blackened and the lover's statement has been proven true
> because the doubt has vanished and doubtlessness is established, therefore I, devoid of qualities, dance.

The contiguity between the *khwaja* and the hijra, who both meet at the point of the *sadaa suhaagan*, would explain why so many men would come to Jaina and ask her to breathe on a small vessel of water after reading the Qur'an. Upon inquiring, Jaina would say, "His wife is pregnant and ill. So that her health and the baby's health is not harmed, and to ensure everything happens smoothly, they will take the water and cook their dinner with it." Apart from having the power of *barakat* (beatitude), Jaina made her living by making garlands of flowers, and only her garlands were allowed in the *mazar*. The *khwaja* and the hijra in their turning away from the world into a formless future, which some would call liberation, point out the inevitable failure of the social in organizing bodies, anatomies, and most of all the carnal. The tomb of the *khwaja*, the fruit and leaves growing out of the carcasses of hijras and out of Malinowski's sibling-lovers, make fertile grounds for the social to sustain itself. Sexual pedagogy makes apparent the uncertainty of the world and the contradictions the social harbors within it; the alternative to this meaning- and value-giving game is a formless future—which for the *khwaja* is liberation and consummation with God, whereas hijras find their liberation in fucking and in consummating with everyone who might be seduced.

UNBEARABLE DESIRES

I was confused as to what the embryo that had been shat out was supposed to commemorate; perhaps the loss of Jaina's virginity, the passion that her youth and beauty had generated in men, or how close she had come to becoming a woman. Trawick renders the structure of kinship as one of longing: the father's longing for continuity and the son's longing for independence; the daughter's longing for continuity and the mother's longing for independence; the siblings' longing for each other, which must be denied; and the spousal longing for an impossible resolution: "With their various longings, [people support] the continuation of the kinship ideal by investing their different personal dreams in it, but in that very process pulling against each other, making the possibility of each other's total fulfillment all the more remote. As long as this ideal answers to the desires that have been written in their bodies since childhood, they will keep reaching for it, and as long as they reach, its various imperfect manifestations will continue to be born."[20] Perpetuity can only be achieved through the failure of fulfillment, but in that failure, resolution is reconfigured. In Trawick's ethnography, the cross-cousin marriage transfigures the relationship through the consummation of their children's marriage; incest is allowed, but only after spatial and temporal deferral have attenuated its poison into something correct and restorative. If the failures of fulfillment guarantee perpetuity within the house, then what was being guaranteed by the failures outside, in the fucking fields, with all the dead fetuses littered about?

Furthermore, what can we make of their sense of coming very close to a threshold that they could not cross, or were just at the cusp of achieving—the impossible—despite overwhelming skepticism? Lovely almost believed she was pregnant. Jaina was pregnant but couldn't bear it, just like the hijras in the Reddy and Nanda versions of the myth, who came even closer to childbirth than Jaina but were tricked by the *khwaja*. They did not ask for the child to be born, just that they have one in their stomach. The fact that hijras died in all the versions, and that in the version recited by Akhtari the lover lives on and marries a woman, denies the hijra and her lover the legendary status of those couples who died because they loved each other, withering in the unrelenting landscape of domesticity and the violence of the social. What do we make of the unbearability of this kinship in which neither the hijra nor the baby survives the world? What can we make of this form of love that cannot survive visibility and valuation, that fails to resolve itself either in domesticity or in death, that does not flower or fructify? And that, ultimately, leaves behind nothing but the residues of desire itself? Desires might very well be impossible, but unfortunately that is hardly a discouragement from their being carnalized. So, what do we make of the carnal that, in the flames of desire, is allowed to come close to fulfillment? Does the social, in mediating the carnal, in creating the human or taming the animal, chafe in such a way that coy invitations—even as minute and subtle as a glance—can spark an inferno?

The men, too, were obsessed with a hijra's reproductive capabilities. Whenever Lovely, the beautiful hijra, would come to Jaina's flower shop in Bhadrak while waiting for her train to Jajpur, she created a *hungama* (pandemonium) with her spangled sari revealing her breasts and the inviting sway of her hips as she walked. The men would smile and stare with lustful desire in their eyes. Jaina would not help matters by screaming loudly through the market, to Lovely's embarrassed amusement, "Come, someone buy her for tonight; 700 rupees for one night." The men did not ask Lovely directly but would come to Jaina. Especially the barber, where I would get a shave, would ask Jaina, "Can she give birth? Can she get pregnant?" (*Baccha kar sakti hai kya?*). Whenever a particularly feminine and womanly young hijra would appear in the public places, the boys and the familiar hijras would embark on a long conversation on whether she had got herself operated on, whether that operation also meant she could now give birth to babies, and how that was possible. I find both the men's inquiries and the hijras' answers interesting. The fact that the question was asked would allow hijras to say, "Yes, of course, she can, the doctors in Calcutta, Delhi, Bombay can do all this now." If Jaina was asked this question, her answers would vary depending on her mood: when she was flirty and not tired, hijras would sometimes be able to give birth ("Of course, she can, why don't you try? Come tonight, you can see for yourself"), but when she was cross and sleepy the answer would rob hijras of the miraculous operation that would allow them to give birth ("No, how will she give birth, you mad fucker?"). The questions would then focus on whether she could get penetrated, the answer to which would always be yes.

What does this encounter, consisting of questions repeatedly asked in the face of all evidence to the contrary, tell us about how these statements about the babies are being received? The men know that hijras cannot give birth; so then, why do *they* hold on to the hope? Does their persistence show that perhaps they could one day achieve the impossible goal with the help of doctors in large cities, to actualize a miracle similar to the one performed by the Khwaja Garib Nawaz (Chishti), recounted in Akhtari's story? What, then, is being heard in the repeated references to this phantom baby? What can we make of the laughter that ensues? What of the serious questions asked, not just out of curiosity? Even when they receive misleading answers, the questions do not go away; they emerge once again at the appearance of a beautiful new face, or an old familiar face looking beautiful at the moment. If repetition belies the impossibility of choice, then the anxiety that the persistently asked question signals is one that Jaina has already mentioned— men require *din-duniya*. No matter how beautiful a hijra is, she cannot give them children, just terror and beauty. Hijras, with their laughter and unbearability, signal the same social anxiety that is drawn upon by the satirist as described by Siegel: "Buddha negated the value of empirical existence, of family, society, and self, for the sake of liberation from the world of life and death. His negation was an affirmation of the possibility of liberation, of the great joy of extinction. The satirist on the other hand affirms the value and necessity of social, domestic, and personal interaction. His liberation is *in* and not *from* the world."[21] Both, men and hijras, want to have babies; they unfortunately can't have them with each other. This incongruence is the scratching of the social against the carnal, felt in the wistful repetitions, sympathetic clucking, resulting in the never-ending violent play between the human and the animal, manifesting in the idea of the sex drive and excused in the idea of instinct. Ironically, the affirmation of the social and the resolution comes from this wild sex: the satirist, the hijra, like Jaina, tells her lover, "You have to set up your house, *din-duniya*"; that is where liberation is, otherwise one becomes an ascetic, a hijra facing a formless future, the "great joy of extinction," the pleasures of castration. The difference in the two forms of liberation also offers a resolution to the impossible desires, the inevitable failure; the threat of the animal, like the risk of incest, is attenuated through temporal and spatial deferral.

One day Jaina and I ran into an old man. As he hobbled along, leaning on his stick, he called Jaina away for five minutes, whispered something into her ear, and went away. I asked Jaina who he was and what he wanted. She said, "Oh, his name is Ghaffoor Babu, he is the grandfather of that man who came yesterday to your hut." The conversation continued:

> I said, "Oh, what was he saying? Was he asking you to not do *kaam* [fuck] his grandson?"
> Jaina laughed and said, "He might be walking with a stick, but he himself is ever ready to fuck."
> "Have you ever fucked him?"
> Jaina: "Yes, when we were both young; now I am scared by the way he is out of breath that he will die fucking me."
> "You've fucked him *and* his grandson?"
> Jaina: "I've fucked his younger brother, both his sons, and two of his grandsons."

This is not what I had in mind, I will confess, when I began collecting narratives of love affairs, and was a bit gobsmacked by this largesse that didn't pay any heed to laws of incest. When I finally undertook the daunting task of drawing kinship charts, I discovered that Jaina, Shamsheri, Azgari, Akhtari, Mehraj, and Mangu had between them fucked generations of men. Perhaps this is the sweet sad resolution of repeated failures of fertility, repeated attempts that fuel the play between failure and hope, animal and human, nature and culture, the social and its carnality through sons and grandsons—an allegory of survivability.

There is a limit even to this form of liberation, within the larger arch of temporality against which not even babies can provide any respite. Siegel notes, "One function of social satire is the establishment of such secret groups, such refuges in which both hostility and despair are aligned with pleasure. But the pleasure cannot hold. The refusal to suffer cannot last. Satire is painful comedy. There is a sadness intrinsic to it, the sorrow of all transience. When the laughter ceases, as it inevitably must, the circle disappears and those who have laughed realize that they are inextricably a part of the decaying world at which they have looked in amused indignation, a world that will devour them and absorb their laughter."[22] What, then, is happening in the conversations between hijras and men? Scholars have pointed out that "if irony is not always an intentional 'discursive strategy,' its reception cannot be interpreted in straightforward terms of successful comprehension or misfire."[23] To study the reception, then, we turn to Lawrence Cohen's essay, which deals with listening ironically.[24] Even though he is studying senility, the pathology and perversity that the categories of senility and homosexuality entail bring them close enough to warrant a look. Cohen argues that what senility allows is the "radical removal of the voice from culture" because not only does it threaten the cosmic order, the everyday norm, it also "challenges the very continuity of culture." These are also the social threats posed by anal sex, but the laughter, the questions of hijra's reproductivity, the love affairs, the sex in all its pleasurable, erotic, and violent forms, would lead one to believe that unlike the senile voice there are ways the faint strains of hijras and the voices of their lovers remain in culture.

Lest one is accused of romancing this form of fucking, I should clarify that I am trying to point to a sociocultural place where one has not escaped the pathologies, the perversity, the impossibilities of trying to become pregnant through anal sex, but where one has to a certain extent found ways to sidestep them, even if it is only for varying periods of time that all come to an end eventually—because the rectum is a grave, no matter how much it is referred to as a pussy, as all hijras did. Cohen, in his analysis of the documentary film *Complaints of a Dutiful Daughter* (1994), writes that the filmmaker Deborah Hoffmann, by freeing her Alzheimer's-afflicted mother from their shared history, allows her to once again become coherent and cleaves the present from its history. This is what Cohen calls the "ironic time of *now*"; in its reach "beyond expected correspondences, unexpected recognitions occur." One can make a similar argument with regard to the statements of hijras about their babies; men's laughter, the fucking, their inquiries about the possibilities of pregnancy amongst hijras remove the body from its history, and for a moment the rectum does become the vagina and for a moment the semen does fertilize a doomed fetus. Men, too, by the way, sometimes provoke laughter and coax hijras into bed: "I will [gesture fucking with hand] so hard that you will be sent to the hospital"; "I can do it so hard that I can impregnate you."

Cohen writes of this ironic temporality: "Since within it words neither correspond to the expected referents of a shared history (that is, are coherent) nor are they necessarily radically beyond coherence. Senility heard ironically offers no redemptive or hidden speech, but neither does it of necessity reduce the voice to *pralapa* [babble]" (127). Rather than placing the burden of subversion or redemption—or resistance and reinscription—on these dramatic and ironic utterances of hijras, we might read them as a way of giving meaning, however unstable, to a certain form of fucking and responding to a longing for everlasting love and fulfillment that you cannot get anywhere, which in turn is indicative of the pulls of the carnal, the animal, against the disciplines of the social, the cultural, and the draining domestic. "To hear ironically is to hear language and its correspondence and everyday work in unexpected ways" (132). That is why a hijra can get impregnated every day and by several men; every day she might shit out fetuses and get new ones.

RASA

Following Geertz, let us call this form of conversation—this laughter, flirting, sympathetic clucking over a hijra's incapability to produce babies—etiquette. Geertz uses this word to understand the ritualization of interaction between people marking various similarities and differences to counter the unpleasantness, shocks, and realities of the world with an order that brings in predictability, politeness, and art—in other words, a certain aestheticization of everyday life. For our purposes here, however, not etiquette but *rasa*, a concept enacted by the Javanese, which Geertz analyzes as etiquette, is more important. One of Geertz's informants helpfully clarifies this for us:

What is the aim of life? (The informant, a teacher-leader [guru] of a mystic sect, was giving me a kind catechism of his group's beliefs.) The aim of life is to seek emotional peace; other than that there isn't any. No one seeks upset, disturbance; everyone just seeks peace. Now each person starts out on this search for inward peace with a certain amount of capital, as in the market, only it is not in the form of money but of rasa. This capital is neither more nor less than the ability to make other people feel at peace. . . . Every person has a capital of rasa to accomplish this. When I came to his house he emerged in proper style to meet me. This was his capital because it put me at ease; and so I was in turn polite to him, and so he was at ease and his capital of rasa increased. You often see written and hung in people's houses, or hear people say: "Men must have etiquette-feeling (*rasa sopan-santun*)." This etiquette-feeling, this form of politeness, is a kind of instrument or tool for making others peaceful within, and thus yourself also; a kind of capital of rasa, because all movement is from rasa and so this politeness has rasa. If you meet a man on the street and you coast by and don't say, "Where are you going, Pak?" in high-Javanese [the typical Javanese greeting], he will feel upset; and later his upsetness will react back and you will feel upset.[25]

Geertz, charting the topography of *prijaji* religious life, connects etiquette with art and mystical practice: the implication of this connection can bring us closer to the meaning of life or, in other words, to the ethics of conducting a life aesthetically or, in still other words, the ethics of corporealizing a life through *rasa*. Aaron Goodfellow studies Geertz's notion of etiquette and shows how etiquette allows relationships to congeal despite the resistance of language—or more precisely, of kinship terminologies—to accommodate them in an easy fashion: "Displaying such etiquette is both a matter of language and behavior, since it is brought about through the use of words and rests on the linguistic expression of a formality or on actively using language to index specific formal structures and positioning the speaker and the addressee within their frames of reference." He then points to "the force of such etiquette, one that respects, while refusing, the capacity of kin terms and kin grammars to obstruct the life of relationships by obscuring their expression."[26]

The situation of hijras in Odisha can be studied in a similar fashion, but I do not think respect and refusal describe their statements concerning their babies; instead, one can view their statements as the futility of hoping for a baby, while still—nonetheless (or inevitably)—relying on the language of pregnancy and fruition to allow a relationship to develop between her and her lovers. In other words, the etiquette of hearing flirty statements and seductive invitations and responding to them likewise unmoors the body from biologistic understandings of time and space and leaves it open to the improvisational forms of relationship that might emerge from the play of desire and pleasure along the lines that segregate the carnal from the domestic.

To understand *rasa* as something that protects one from the unpleasantness of the world, let us understand the context of the Sanskrit literary traditions from which it emerges. In his article "The Social Aesthetic and Sanskrit Literary Theory," Sheldon Pollock argues, "The broader history of Sanskrit literary culture—we saw precisely this in the history of the idea of *rasabhasa*—fully testifies to a progress, slow but certain, in the elimination of core varieties of conflict, a gradual retreat to an ever more complete disengagement from the world of life's unpleasant realities, in favor of a single moral vision. In literature if not in life, as Bhoja says, 'it must be the good guy, not the bad guy, who wins'."[27] The text is where the passions are a virtue, not something that inhibits one's life plans. The indifference of commentators to the "social-and-moral imagination of Sanskrit literary texts" is a consequence of "the social and the moral as forming a unified sphere of knowledge in premodern India" (197).

Thus, if the text is supposed to make heroes of its readers, its heroes themselves must be morally upright. This in turn means that the passion or *rasa* of the text cannot be generated through desiring improper objects, which leads both authors and readers into a quandary; how would you then account for the desire of the villain, whom the hero will eventually slay, but who, in order to make the hero heroic, must equal him in all respects, in *rasa*? That is why the *rasas*—or passion itself—cannot be inappropriate; the words of the villain exhorting his love are as tasteful as the *rasa* of the hero for the heroine, but it is the object of his affection that is inappropriate. Both author and reader must acknowledge the validity of the villain's desire but also recognize it as being morally wrong, and this is done by disaggregating the text and emphasizing it differently at different moments. The reader acknowledges the *rasa* of the character but remembers in the end that he must not be like the villain, desiring the improper object, but must rather be like the hero. This lesson is an important one because it allows for the sacred to absorb the profane, even if for a short duration, and explains to us the space created in time by hijra laughter and seduction. A hijra's passion and desire get a response—acknowledgment and recognition that more often than not are also actualized in sex—but in the end, the laughter must die only to be renewed somewhere else, at some other time.

Pollock traces how the language of the hero and the villain must be the same in its *rasa* but aimed at two opposite ends—moral and immoral. The two forms of writing that emerged, the rasa and the *rasabhasa*, are similar in their aesthetic sensibilities but differ in their goals. That is when the responsibility for recognizing the passion, but also its inappropriateness, was divided and placed equally on the text and the *rasika*, the knowing reader. Pollock writes:

> If propriety lies at the heart of *rasa*, rasa becomes the heart of a moral economy of literature. It can produce its effects only to the degree that the imaginative discourse represents, and thereby inevitably serves to reproduce, what is appropriate to a given situation, which in turn is intelligible only in terms of a unified vision of the social order. Thus when one learns what literature is, how it works and when one learns to be a good reader, a *rasika* or a *sahrdaya*, one is learning what is normative in the everyday world. To produce readers of Sanskrit literature is to produce certain kinds of social subjectivities. *Rasabhasa* and the *anaucitya* that provides its logic are the locus where criticism of literary form and criticism of literary representation—criticism of life—intersect. (215)

The text and certain kinds of speech, like flirting, must then have a larger point (*mahavakyartha*) that works through the aesthetic of suggestion, which the reader with an "innate receptivity" (*upahitasamskara*) can understand. This understanding must then be measured in terms of right and wrong that emerge from yet another shared realm of meaning that includes both the reader and the text.

When we return to our scene of evenings spent in the teashops with hijras regaling everybody with laughter—the *hasya rasa* that leads to an erotic relationship between her and her lover, the *sringara rasa*—it would make sense to read the drama, pace Pollock, disaggregately.[28] The statements and the desire for a baby in the myth is the desire for moral validation that will recognize the relationship of desire as one of love as well, the rectum as the womb, *rasabhasa* as *rasa*. Even when dead, the baby is an attempt toward that, but bears the temporal marking of that relationship; it is born, like any other baby, but it cannot survive like the ones to the manor born. The relationship between the *rasa* and the *rasika*, the hijra and her lover, the character and the reader can, in Pollock's words, theoretically be regarded in three dimensions: as a dimension of a textual object, as a competence of a reader-subject, and as a transaction between the two: "It is a process that exists as totality even while its moments can be analytically disaggregated, and it is this analytical disaggregation—or rather the different emphases that such disaggregation permits—that marks and makes the history of Indian thinking on the subject" (209–10). Such transactions are only possible if the reader and the text, the listener and the speaker, both inhabit a common realm of meaning. Pollock gives an example of this in the following poem:

It is a very heavy water jug I'm carrying,
my friend, and I've come back quickly.
I've got to rest a second since I'm weak
and sweating and sighing from exhaustion.

He then comments, "Now, it is perfectly true that what makes it possible for the sensitive reader to understand that this verse is about 'concealing stolen love-making,' as Mammata puts it, is the 'specificity of the speaker.' But the only thing that allows us to specify this specificity is the reader's participation in and acceptance of a particular universe of social meaning as made available in the texts of a literary culture" (206–7). This is how the boy in the shop understood Shamsheri's invitations to fuck; this is how a lot of men understand hijras' coquetry.

SUKH DUKH: TRANSACTIONS IN LAUGHTER AND PAIN

The transactions between hijras and their lovers follow in similar ways: the laughter is important because it makes life in Bhadrak, one of the poorest districts in India, bearable; it is a transaction of *sukh dukh* (happiness and sadness). Once when a child not yet in his teens was staring at Jaina's breasts with a lot of hunger, she lifted her lungi to flash the seductive darkness of the region between her legs and screamed, "Come fuck me." I started laughing uncontrollably, but Amrita told me not to encourage Jaina.[29] Later I asked Jaina, Akhtari, and Shamsheri, "Why do you always talk like that? Why do you do that?" Jaina responded, "I try to make everybody laugh, even you, who have come here, far away from your *mulk* (land). You must feel strange here; by laughing, the heart becomes light. These men, they come to me to talk, they share their *sukh dukh* and their problems and I try to make them laugh and make their *ji halka*" (heart/chest/soul lighten). *Ji ghabrana* is when the heart beats fast because anxiety and worry have gripped it in the face of problems one cannot surmount, and in Bhadrak there were problems aplenty: the external conditions of structural poverty in all its guises, consequences, and effects were present. Men were forever signaling Jaina and the other hijras to come aside, and animated whispering would take place between them; when asked about the surreptitious conversation, Jaina would tell me—in confidence, of course—what the man said about the problems he was facing.

Laughter (*hasya*, one of the *sthayibhava* of *sringara*)[30] that makes the *ji halka* was a form of care that hijras offered; the references to the baby and the fucking would arouse the men and would both reveal the pleasure of desiring and result in the pleasure of being desired in men that were scarcely desired in the world next door. It is this form of sharing *sukh dukh* and making the *ji halka*, allowing the burden of life to be borne by beautiful men, and sometimes resulting in love—a love manifested through the feeling of being pregnant, of carrying its moral witness, which is the baby. The baby would by its very existence and likeness, dead or alive, transform a hijra into an appropriate object of desire—a woman. Hijras, through their theatricality, inherit a form of aesthetics that, I have argued, can be read as *rasa*. *Rasa* is the making present of an emotion when it is not an experience that one has gone through; this aestheticization of the everyday through *sringara* helps form a buffer against the world.

What form of caring is enacted by the sharing of *sukh dukh* and by associating the laughter and the fucking? It is not the economy of creation and destruction but rather, I would argue, the action of preservation, of sustaining and sustenance. Looking at the care afforded by the erotic relationships of hijras through the eyes of preservation—or more accurately of sustenance—would allow hijras to enter the economy of life diagonally. She is bent or *banka*. *Rasa*, as Geertz and Pollock have studied it, preserves us from the despair of this transient world; it is what triangulates and makes possible the economy of creation and destruction. It is also the form of care taken up by the *sadaa suhaagan* who implores passionately for a child to be given to the barren woman. *Sadaa suhaagan* cannot produce children or family, and like Jaina she doesn't destroy the possibility of the householder in men. This form of care sends the lover to his wife, asks Allah to give the child to the woman, blesses the child and the woman with prosperity, fertility, and fortune to make her life bearable in the world, while opting out of these projects at the same time. The care that makes the *ji halka* cannot remove or solve the problems of the world, but it fortifies its inhabitants to bear life's knocks once again. The men would speak of the carnality of the fucking in explicitly constitutional ways: "There was so much heat built up in my body, *kaam karne ke baad* [doing work/fucking], the body has turned calm." The anxieties of the world, the heat generated through desire, all of this was calmed by the fucking.

The sharing of the *sukh dukh* allows her to partake in the world in a certain way. This is what qualifies as her renunciation, her diagonal entrance into the economy; she is neither inside nor outside the home and the world but lives beside it. This also explains the laughter, the irony. Siegel, in his study of the laughter of Krishna, an avatar of Vishnu the preserver, writes:

> Within the history of religion of Krishna there has been a dialectic at work between the theologian and the comedian, one that balances the god and creates an invigorating tension. The theologian, stressing the absolute divinity of Krishna, makes the god serious; the comedian emphasizing the absolute humanness of Krishna, makes the cowherd funny. The more divinely serious he becomes, however, the greater his potential for comedy, for comic revelations of his humanness; conversely the more comic he is, the greater his appeal, the greater his potential for being taken seriously. Comedy vitalizes, then, the very devotion of which it makes fun. It preserves what it seems to destroy.[31]

The rectum then might be the grave, but the semen it ingests is an accursed share, its death inevitable.

Hijras' experience of physical space, interestingly, is congruent with her being beside the world. For example, Jaina lives in a brick-walled single room that is attached to the house where her mother, brothers, their wives, and their children all live. The house is half-constructed, with two floors, and the rooms have been divided among three brothers with separate kitchens. Jaina's room shares its back wall with the left-hand side wall of the house, but you enter it separately from the street. There is no door that connects the room with the house, but they share a wall; they are attached. This affords Jaina all the privacy she needs to entertain her lovers, allowing the family and Jaina to live under the salubrious condition of being blind to and cultivating obliviousness to what is going on under their noses. This spatial arrangement allows me to extend the metaphor of how hijras live beside the household and the economy of the world and participate in it sideways. It also explains the necessity of a hijra's presence when there is a wedding or a baby born; they are neither bride nor groom, neither father nor mother, but their blessings are sought precisely for those occasions, events that they have opted out of. To understand the dynamics, limits, and possibilities of endurance, sustenance, perseverance, and preservation—and how fucking sustains both hijras and their lovers—I once again rely on *rasa* and how it is used in a text that predates all the texts that Pollock treats in his article: the *Bhagwata Purana* (c. eighth–tenth centuries).

The plenitude celebrated by hijras in the form of blessing other people's babies and marriages, through which they earn their living and materially sustain their existence, gets related to the laughter and fucking through the myth retold by Akhtari: she reads a myth of fertility-bestowing fruits and shrines as one emerging from a love story failed by the world; the connection is offered through *rasa*. The fertility-granting and the sexual pedagogy that hijras instantiate alleviate the cruelties of the world and of domesticity that result in *ji ghabrana*. Let us reexamine *rasa* to understand the various ways in which its dynamics and economics allow for the sharing of *sukh dukh*. The first lines from the *Bhagwata Purana* that I want to address are as follows: "My dear gopis, what auspicious activities must the flute have performed to enjoy the nectar of Krishna's lips independently and leave only a taste for us gopis for whom that nectar is actually meant! The forefathers of the flute, the bamboo trees, shed tears of pleasure. His mother, the river on whose bank the bamboo was born, feels jubilation, and therefore her blooming lotus flowers are standing like hair on her body."[32]

The nectar of Krishna's lips is being savored by the bamboo flute, while the *gopis* are tasting the *rasa* through mediations of sound and songs. Krishna's nectar or *rasa* here keeps on expanding exponentially to give pleasure first to the bamboo flute, then the *gopis* who are listening to the music, the trees who feel pleasure to see one of their own being held to Krishna's lips, and the river that feels pleasure because her water sustained the bamboo that made the flute that Krishna has taken to his lips. One can juxtapose with this scene of conjugal bliss between Krishna and the flute the scene where the baby born between a man and a woman is being blessed by hijras, who are celebrating the occasion along with the whole family. Thus the nectar (semen) of the man, even though it is produced by him and consumed by his flute (family), seems to be tasted by everybody around him. Hijras, too, can be seen to share and taste the pleasures of fertility and reproduction when they come to auspicious occasions and participate in the magical expansion of the man's nectar. When I used to walk the streets of Bhawanipatna with Damru, Nandita, Pawan Hijra, Ghungi, and the others, men would always stop us and ask us to come bless the opening of their new shop, a wedding, the birth of a baby. This struck me as odd, since in the urban areas of Calcutta, Delhi, and Bombay, while the presence of hijras was considered inevitable on certain occasions, their ritualized appearances were often viewed with fear and dread, given their tendencies to extort money and not back down from a fight. These invitations to participate can be understood through the necessity of their presence to help expand the nectar of the man by tasting it in various ways and forms.

The complementarity between men and the world is a bit nauseating, given that its purpose is to sustain the conceit of masculinity regarding their powerful nectar/semen—semen that the boys in Bhadrak would never stop praising as something that would not only make hijras pregnant, but pregnant like dogs with four or six babies. The statements about the babies transfigure fucking into caring precisely because it makes his semen magical if it can result in embryos in the rectum, one might argue. Reading semen, nectar, and *rasa* as one helps make sense of the various statements heard in the marketplace of Bhadrak, where men would say how they fucked their wives twelve times and needed to fuck more; how they would need to fuck at least four times every night and would keep on fucking for hours and hours until hijras would break out in sweat or the poor woman would pass out with exhaustion. Hijras in praising and desiring the virility/strength/ prowess of the penis, calling it a *hathiyar* (weapon), not only eroticized the violence of it but also preserved it as "phallus and penis and signifier and gender and god"; in castrating themselves, and seducing the penis to dispense its precious nectar, they also destroy it.[33]

Since the bamboo trees in the lines of the *purana* are not explicitly labeled as the flute's fathers, there is yet another equally valid and much more palatable explanation given by Sanatana Gosvami. He explains that the trees are weeping not tears of joy but tears of unhappiness, because they themselves are not being held at Krishna's lips. His explanation continues: "One may object that the trees in Vrindavana should not lament for that which is impossible for them to obtain, just as a beggar certainly doesn't lament because he is forbidden to meet the king. But the trees are actually just like intelligent persons who suffer when they cannot obtain the goal of life. Thus the trees are crying because they cannot get the nectar of Krishna's lips." The lines recognize through lament that they could not achieve their life's goal, which was the nectar of Krishna's lips. The ambiguity embedded in these lines is reflected in a hijra's position when she celebrates the newborn child, an event mottled with the sadness of knowing that the babies will never be her own but are at least her lover's.

The second passage I want to treat reads as follows:

> With their flowing waves—the deep rivers drenched their banks,
> making them damp and muddy.
> Thus the rays of the sun, which were as fierce as poison,
> could not evaporate the earth's *rasa* or parch its green grass.[34]

The *purana* later describes the sun: "The sun with its annihilating form can drink up with its terrible rays all the water of the ocean, of living bodies, and of the earth itself without giving anything in return."[35] And when the sun is not taking on such an annihilating form, but is fierce, then it is the rivers who drench their banks and give *rasa* to the earth, sustaining life. Focusing on this line might reiterate the earlier point made already about *rasa*, one that preserves one from the exposure to the poisonous sunrays, but it leads us to the question of whether hijras should be seen as one of the many characters that enable the incompetent if not impotent family to reproduce itself. Or do we read in her caring and providing sustenance a certain criticism of the poisonous world, which is ever threatening to annihilate everything? This caring undoes hijras themselves and forces them to enter the protocols of the world to sustain the very households from which they escape. Does the form of the hijra's care result in a certain temporal existence in which she becomes a virgin every night—like the waters on a bank that flow continuously—each lapping wave providing sustenance and refreshing the earth?

CONCLUSION

Even a brief look at the great epic the *Mahabharata* will reveal that sexual reproduction to ensure continuity, perpetuity, and futurity is extremely difficult between a man and his wife and involves the participation of a whole host of personalities that emerge from the margins to contribute to the success of the grand event. The epic details three generations of a dynasty that had produced heirs from everywhere and everybody except the husband of the woman. Ambika and Ambalika, wives of Vicitravirya, after his death, sleep with Vyasa, the author of the epic, to beget Dhrtrastra and Pandu. Vyasa was incidentally begotten by the women's mother-in-law, Satyavati, through the sage Parasar, not her husband. Thus, the half-brother inseminates the fields owned by the king. The two sons produced heirs through difficulty themselves and through ready help given to them by gods. Kunti produced five sons with the help of Indra, Dharma, Vayu, and the two Asvins—as her husband was cursed to die if he touched his queen.

Doniger studies these myths and the laws of the *Manushastra* to make a point about the ever-expanding boundaries of Hindu marriage. She comments, "Hovering on the borders of legitimate marriage to define it by demonstrating what it is not, adultery and the *niyoga* (levirate) together demonstrate that Hindu marriage is, in itself, an elusive institution caught between a rock and a hard place."[36] The earlier point I made about resemblance is important because if the son/crop that grows in the woman/field owned by one's brother, then the child has to resemble the owner of the field, the husband; he will be the father, not the one who spilt his seed. If the child resembles not the owner but the man who generously gave his seed, then this would undo the leviratic contract at least as mentioned in the *Mansushastra*. This sexual act, in Doniger's argument, not only shows how biology is unmoored when the aim is to sustain the social, but also how a space in time is created for laws to be suspended precisely so that they can then sustain themselves. A space is created by the sacred for profaning that consolidates it, which it accommodates to handle the insufficiencies of the family to reproduce itself. These are what gods and sages did in times long ago, and I want to argue that this is what a hijra does as well. She obviously does not beget heirs, but her form of loving and fucking allow for laughter and for the sharing of *sukh dukh*, making the *ji halka*; in other words, she provides relief from the maddening illusions of the world, the abrasive social, and the deceptively comforting shelter of domesticity. The failure to reproduce is also obviously felt acutely by cis women when they suffer from deaths of infants and miscarriages or just fail to get pregnant. In rural Odisha this resulted in a recognition of "mutual fatedness" between hijras and cis women of the settlement and further points to similarities created by conditions of poverty amongst bodies even though they might be different through the vectors of gender.[37] Thus, the context of poverty can be seen to change the coordinates for queer theory in quite fundamental ways.

In this chapter, I have shown that the various ways and forms of life that hijras inhabit are both within the larger Hindu and Muslim universe of sociality and outside it—a posture I describe as being diagonal to that world. This position is implicated under a larger rubric of endurance or preservation in the following ways. The first involves a type of ironic speech that is geared toward producing the aesthetic emotion of *sringara*—love with laughter as its main foundation (*sthayi bhava*), but with swirling moods of melancholia, hope, sadness, and euphoria surrounding it. Second, I show how the frequent talk of "babies" allows an impossible desire to find expression in the world, even if the protagonists are doomed to die; that expression here is anchored in a shared symbolic universe of myth and ritual available in such figures as the *sada suhagaan* and the permutations of asceticism and eroticism that the various actors inhabit. Third, the forms of sociality engendered through sex have the double movement of taking away the male from the world of domesticity and returning him to it more fortified to meet the demands of domesticity. Fourth, I argue that hijras offer the world a mode of care that is recognized at both collective and individual levels in the acts of blessing that are particularly efficacious for the fruition of sexual and reproductive desires that are embedded in the world of domesticity.

Finally, Siegel wrote of laughter, "Comedy can be refuge, if not redemption; its laughter can be solace, if not release."[38] So, likewise, hijras' fucking can offer respite while running the risk of rendering one a hijra ascetic as well; but there is a limit to this relief, and it comes in the figure of the fetuses that hijras shit in the fucking fields. While desires might be resolved through the lover's son and grandson as she is impregnated every evening, a hijra's repeated enactments of love, in ceaseless waves, can result in a very melancholic experience of temporality with no liberation in sight. But at least there is laughter and fucking.

2

IN FALSE BROTHERS, EVIL AWAKENS

Given that hijras rarely become householders, their role within the family is almost never that of husband or father. As hijras grow older, their relationship to the family is no longer mediated through fathers but instead through brothers, when the latter replace their fathers as heads of households. We can picture their movement over time, across the web of kinship, as diagonal; they remain brothers and sons, but become transformed into uncles as their own brothers turn into householders and have children. This chapter studies how hijras—even when caught in the web of kinship—maintain forms of relatedness that defamiliarize notions of asceticism and participation in kinship.

THE LAND BELONGS TO THE FUTURE

Jaina had been working since she was ten years old. Her former jobs included milking cows for a Marwari cow trader, employment in two biscuit factories in the neighboring district of Baripada, and laboring in construction. She was also a cook in a small roadside eatery, where she made meals for migrant workers. After working for fifty-odd years and helping her mother raise her two brothers and two sisters, she returned to Bhadrak in 2006 to a room from which she sold small quantities of spices. She also ran a small flower shop, where she made garlands for nearby mosques and mazars. Although her flower shop was to be demolished to make room for bigger shops, Jaina was unfazed because she could no longer afford the flowers, which came from Calcutta, to make garlands anyway; floods had destroyed a lot of flowers in the last Ramzaan (August 2010), the month in which Jaina would have earned the most. Because she had a place to stay and took her meals with her brother, she was only mildly disappointed by these turns of events, which might have worried other shopkeepers far more. I asked her why she still peddled spices and flowers when both jobs were obviously not going well. She replied, "I can't ask my brothers for money every day. They might give me money some days, but they will start complaining afterward. I can't ask money for every little thing I need, plus the money I give to Muneeza"—referring to her brother's third child, four years old, who would come every hour repeatedly pleading with Jaina to give money for small snacks.

This sense of awareness Jaina had about the limits and possibilities of kinship with her brothers made me prick up my ears because, right at the beginning of my fieldwork in 2008, she had claimed that her brothers loved her, as did everyone in the family. "You eat here every day," she stated. "You tell me—can't you see how much they love me? They never insult me, and when I am ill they buy me medicines." This attestation had led me—mistakenly—to frame the relationship between hijras and their families in terms of either acceptance or ostracism—triumphs of either filial love or family honor. While Jaina claimed that there was affection, she was also aware that she could not completely depend on her brothers to fund the small luxuries that arose daily. She feared that she would then become vulnerable to her brothers' accusations of sponging money while giving nothing in return. The restraint exercised in not asking for money every day and the love that was proudly claimed revealed a certain tension between the brothers that hijras were hard-pressed to negotiate, since they had not exactly remained "a brother." This form of calibrating transactions of money and food at home to maintain amicable relationships and a pleasant atmosphere was also observable in other spaces and times, in which other types of transactions took place.

For example, Jaina's brothers would never come to visit her shop or the shops of her friends because raunchy conversations about fucking and cocks abounded in those spaces. Their presence, Jaina told me, would markedly change the atmosphere, and nobody would be able to tease and flirt freely. "Wouldn't you feel ashamed to talk about fucking and touching men in front of your family members?" she asked. I replied in the affirmative. "So, why are you asking such stupid questions—like why don't your brothers come here? I have told them that they shouldn't say salaam to me or even talk to me in public. Whatever they need to say can wait until I am home. If people get to know that they are related to me, people can point fingers at them as well. People will tease them by saying, 'Oh your brother is a *maichiya*, she fucks so many men. I don't want my brothers to feel ashamed because of me." But given that everybody, including her brothers, knew that Jaina was a hijra who got fucked by a lot of boys, it seemed that what was at stake was a certain performance of attentiveness that the brothers showed Jaina in keeping away, and thereby allowing her to flirt freely.

One of her brothers, who worked at the post office, often used to tell me, "We all know—even our mother knows—what Jaina's nature is. What to do? Just as Allah has made each of the five fingers of the hand different, Allah has not made everybody the same" [*hum sab jaante hai, Ammi bhi jaanti hai, unka nature kaisa hai, kya karenge aur kya, Jaise Allah pak haath ka paanch ungli ek samaan nahin banaya hai, Allah sab ko ek rakm ka nahin banaya hai*]. The brothers explicitly acknowledged Jaina's desire (to be fucked) as natural but different, just as the thumb is distinct from the four fingers. The presence of a hijra sibling was not seen as a breach of nature so much as a breach of structure. Hijras' not leaving the family, but rather remaining in the household, led to a conundrum that obscured and thus punctuated the movement by which brothers became householders—and who are, by this movement, positioned against each other.

One day when we were returning from a visit to Jaina's widowed sister Jaira Bai, in the neighboring village of Nuasahi, Jaina pointed to a tract of land she had bought thirty years ago: a rectangular piece that stood out because it was the only segment of the large area that remained uncultivated, whereas its four sides were furrowed and the land around it stuffed with paddy. She said, "This belongs to me." I was a bit surprised, never having imagined that she owned anything. She said, "The land is worth six and a half lakhs rupees [650,000 INR], but my brothers are asking me to sell it to them for four lakhs [400,000 INR]." Given that her brothers took care of her, I inquired, why wouldn't she sell it to them? She replied, "They take care of me because they want the land; they will throw me out after I give it to them. I am a hijra. There is nobody in front of me [referring to her lack of children]. When I can no longer work, how will I expect to live? My brothers won't look after me—they will look after their own children. They will not think twice before kicking me out on the streets."

To understand the plaiting of claimed love, calibrations of care, and the suspicions of betrayal that coordinate hijras' relationship with their family, let us look at the two different temporal frames that Jaina inhabited vis-à-vis her family and their enactments of love. The first temporal frame was defined by the tendency toward tenderness on the part of her brothers that took place in the register of the everyday.[1] For instance, they bought medicines when Jaina fell ill, gave her food to eat, took care of her when her business floundered, and more importantly they negotiated public spaces in a way so as to not embarrass Jaina when she flirted. Avoiding her in public was a way to prevent situations from arising in which Jaina might be used as a means of insulting the brothers and the family. When speaking from this temporal frame, Jaina would be proud of the love she claimed and received from her family. The other temporal frame in which Jaina spoke consisted of the transformation of brothers into householders and fathers, marked by the movement of land through inheritance, which was expected to take place in the future but cast its shadow on the present. The materiality of land gave Jaina a language for discussing how the relationship between brothers might corrode over time. These two disparate temporal frames resulted in an everyday context in which the future was already part of the present, thus bringing about conflict by the mixing of tenderness and potential aggression. Jaina was held hostage to the future in the everyday. This made Jaina prudent in her demands of her brothers: she could ask for some help but doing so made her vulnerable to the accusations of sponging off them. Land appeared in this case, both as the imagined cause of her brothers' possible betrayal and, paradoxically, as a point to leverage one's security against that very betrayal.

Shamsheri recounted to me an instance of the tension produced by these two temporal frames—the present and the future—as materialized through land. She told me that around fifteen years ago she was tricked into marriage through *jaadu tona* (magic). Her brother had asked Shamsheri to marry a certain woman, and Shamsheri's mother had also agreed; at the time Shamsheri didn't realize that her brother was marrying her off to *his* kept woman. Every time I asked her why she agreed to the marriage she replied, "Magic was done on me [*Mujh pe jaadu tona hua tha*]." Shamsheri told me:

> She [her now ex-wife] is a prostitute. She eats from a hundred places; how can she eat only from one place? She says so herself. She is so fat. She told me, "You are a mosquito, I am a she-elephant, how can I stay with you?"

In our *dharm*, "when a woman sins, it goes on her man, and when a man sins it goes on his son." She did some magic on me, and with such magic even the jungle's tiger will get trapped.

Azgari, who was fiddling with bicycles nearby, chipped in:

The marriage was done very silently, nobody knew. There were rumors, and when we went to ask Shamsheri, "Listen, we have heard that you are getting married, is it true?" she denied it. Then one day she came with the woman. The next morning Shamsheri came to me [Azgari] and said, "The woman's blouse was wet, I asked her why was it wet and I saw that milk was coming out of her breasts. She told me that she had been pregnant but had aborted the baby [*baccha gira diya*]." Shamsheri continued sleeping next to her mother and the prostitute-wife was so upset that she went around telling everybody in the morning that Shamsheri sleeps next to her mother and does not come to her at night. It was true; she is a hijra, how can she have sex with her—she doesn't have the *hathiyar* (weapon/instrument/penis). It was later that Shamsheri found out that the woman had been sleeping with Shamsheri's brother and continued to do so. When he [Shamsheri's brother] left his concubine after a year or two, she went back to her mother's place. It was then when she filed a lawsuit against Shamsheri for maintenance expenses. When she couldn't pay, the court decided that Shamsheri would stay in jail for six months every year.

At this point, I must mention that Shamsheri, though a practicing Muslim, invoked a particularly Hindu concept of *karta* in which the person who commits the sin puts at stake not only one's own life but also the lives of people one is related to through duties of expiation.[2] A vast scholarship has shown that the everyday lived reality of South Asia is characterized by the interweaving of Islamic and Hindu ideas and concepts. Hijras stand as particular examples of such interweaving, and I have sought to privilege the way they have used terms and concepts to show their absorption and embeddedness in both the Hindu and the Muslim worlds of rural Odisha.

Shamsheri got help with freeing herself from the lawsuit of maintenance expenses by a community-based organization (CBO) called Santi Seva, made up of sexual minorities at high risk for HIV/AIDS working under a nongovernmental organization (NGO) called the Fellowship Project. She sold the three *katthas* [plot] of land she had inherited from her father, and her mother sold one *kattha* of land that Shamsheri would have inherited after her mother's death.[3] Another day when Shamsheri was recounting—partly to herself, partly to me—how her brother betrayed her, she suddenly whispered to me:

> I have been paying the property taxes for the two katthas of land for my mother for the last thirty years, but in my name.[4] Since I have taken care of my mother all these years, I will make sure she testifies in the courts that the kattha of land she sold was not for my lawsuit but for her food and medications, because the other two boys do not take care of her. This way the other two katthas can come to me and my brothers cannot say that I have already eaten my share. I will take the other two katthas and ruin them. I want to ruin him [the brother whose mistress she had married]. He didn't even come to see me in jail.

Jaina, who was half-dozing nearby, woke up shocked when she heard this and said, "No, don't do that. Let these things be bygones now, live cordially. You are alone, who will take care of you when you are old? If you forgive your brothers then they will take care of you." Shamsheri did not pay heed and gazed out the window. Jaina walked out, fuming and furious. Even I was a bit puzzled by Jaina's insistence on this reconciliatory position. I turned to her, "How can you say 'forgive your brother' when you know what he's done? He coerced Shamsheri to marry a woman he wanted to marry but couldn't, then did not take care of the woman after abandoning her. So many problems resulted in consequence—and when the lawsuit happened he did not even go to the police station?" Jaina said, "No, no she shouldn't look for vengeance." After muttering to herself for a while, she turned to me and said, "You think Shamsheri's brothers don't know she is plotting this against them. Of course they know, this village is not so big—everybody knows what is happening in everybody's house. People have killed each other for so little land"—she stretches out her arms the entire span—"I am scared that they will cut her throat if she does all this. After the mother dies, she will be left all alone. Who cares whether she lives or dies? They will kill her and nothing will happen. She should be careful."

Shamsheri was not upset by the fact that her brother used her for playing the field, nor was she morally troubled that she had taken part in such illegitimacy. What she did mind was that her brother didn't show any concern or tenderness when she was thrown in jail and was being taken to the cleaners by his very own mistress. It was the absence of care at that time that marked the brother's betrayal and compelled Shamsheri to plot against him, scheming to inherit his land. These ethnographic incidents reveal only one aspect of kinship relations that plays out on the substrate of land and the inheritance of property. Shamsheri's brother did not betray her because of land, and neither was Shamsheri planning to betray her brother because she wanted the land for herself, but it was only through land that she was capable of redressing the wrong done to her. Jaina also inadvertently contradicted herself and showed us the grain of fraternal intimacy in kinship when she remarked that Shamsheri's brothers might kill her if they found themselves robbed of land. If brothers can kill each other for land, then why does Jaina think that her brothers love her only for her share of land, when they could take it by murdering her? If land is not the object of the brothers' care and attentiveness toward Jaina, then how can we account for their care? That can hardly be the reason they are attentive toward her. Consequently, why be skeptical of the care afforded to her every day?

MORE THAN KIN, LESS THAN KIND

Land gives expression to kinship relations not only because of the affective intensity it generates but also because of how inheritance of land connects the family with ancestors. This argument runs the risk of reducing land to a purely symbolic language, whereas the materiality and income-generating potential of land, especially in rural-agricultural India, cannot be ignored when one has children for whom one must provide. Nevertheless, the economic value of land cannot be the sole consideration, given that the intensity with which disputes over land are conducted threatens one not only with bankruptcy but also with loss of one's life. In short, if betrayal is an ever-present risk in the general condition of being relational, land provides the vehicle or material for enacting such a desire. It reveals how time and specifically futurity infect the grain of fraternal intimacy.

A large share of the anthropological canon would testify to the relevance of property transmission to kinship. Though land inevitably becomes the ground on which fraternity between hijras and their brothers is staked, it is neither sufficiently the cause of violence nor the result of intimacy.[5] We could draw some support for this argument from Freud's hypothesis in *Totem and Taboo*, specifically the implication that brothers can never fight about who is fucking whom because a fight over that issue would result in a descent into animality and would be a breach of the most fundamental law that gives form not only to the social but to the human.[6] In the aforementioned ethnographic scenes I recounted, ambivalence inherent in kinship gets rerouted through land.[7] Shamsheri attempts to redress the wrongs done by her brother, because of his lack of care, by seeking to rob him of his land. This is a vehicle for inflicting pain, for injuring the other party, oddly enough both in the present and the future. Jaina understood land to be the reason tenderness was afforded to her and why it could be taken away. Shamsheri did not find the fact of her brother's fucking around problematic, nor did Matru, Jaina's brother—it is their nature. But all of them use property rights to fight each other and to remain mindful themselves that all brotherhood is false, that eventually brothers seek out ways to kill each other.

The Indian family drama begins when the father dies and the elder brother takes over the role of the father. Fights over land are proverbial and often deflected through the wives of brothers who refuse to live with each other. Land crystallizes in itself this particular vision of the family drama in the Indian context. Put another way, land and property can be a seen as the literal material for the crystallization of fraternal antagonism, thus the very vehicle for allowing brothers to remain human while fighting like animals in a way that is expected and inevitable.[8] Let me offer, by way of example, a rereading of a legal case analyzed by Oliver Mendelsohn that illustrates the affective aspects of property holding, a case that allowed for killing as well as the exercise of restraint. The property disputes in question were raging between one Jagat Singh and his cousins, beginning with the fragmentation of properties after the death of their great-grandfather. Jagat Singh returned to his ancestral land in 1965 to consolidate his holdings but faced resistance from his cousins, who also claimed legal rights over several properties. Jagat Singh's side of the family had relatively prospered over the generations, and he was educated and far more familiar with the legal system than his cousins. Because the cousins had remained in the village, however, they retained the loyalty of the extended family and sometimes used physical force to take over the properties claimed by Jagat Singh, whereas Jagat Singh had only his son by his side.

Mendelsohn writes, "The inconclusiveness of litigation in relation to the basic conflict is certainly characteristic of litigation over land in India," yet he barely acknowledges the various reasons that contributed to this inconclusiveness and dismisses the position taken by the cousins as faulty.[9] The complex calculations of kinship are barely acknowledged by Mendelsohn when he observes that "family relations are peculiarly 'multiplex' and they often serve to entrench and ramify a dispute beyond the bounds of a similar material conflict between socially more distant people."[10] This is because both residence and affiliation are factors that allow claims over land to be legitimate but do not offer any resolution to disputes that had been raging between the brothers for thirty years. Being related contributes to keeping the conflict alive rather than resolving it, given that claims of ownership made in courts are justified through arguments of lineage and inheritances, while claims of ownership in the village, outside the courts, are consolidated through physical force commanded through the consent of distant and immediate family members.[11]

Mendelsohn offers a portrait of the affective nature of property that does not align clearly with economic interests. He writes, "It can be conceded that a measure of material satisfaction may well have induced Raghbir Singh [the poor cousin] to give up his struggle, at least temporarily. But what incentive would Jagat Singh have had to give up any of his land? For him harmony is a minor value when it is opposed to legitimate self-interest, and his standard of legitimacy is the law of the land. He would have been prepared to make only the most minor concession to his opponents, so minor that it would scarcely have satisfied them."[12] This is the point where I place my argument that hijras, by remaining with their family members, teach us how to create harmony in the face of the antagonistic intimacy of fraternity. Property disputes, I would argue, stem from the condition of fraternity that unfolds over time as a competition between householders.[13] Given that hijras do not have marriages that result in supportive affinal relatives, and since they do not produce sons, alliance actually makes them more vulnerable to fraternal violence as it plays out through land—as exemplified in the case of Jaina. In the remainder of the chapter, I shall demonstrate how hijras intervene in the everyday life of the family, which cannot be seen as acquiescing to the violence of the family but as adhering to a standard of legitimacy that is not necessarily the law of the land but is the logic of sustenance or preservation.

In her analysis of women as witnesses of violence, Veena Das writes how the temporal depth in which one constructs one's subjectivity "may occupy the signs of injury and give them a meaning not only through acts of narration but through the work of repairing relationships and giving recognition to those whom the official norms had condemned." I want to borrow this idea of temporal projections to compare the ways in which Jaina and Shamsheri negotiated land transactions that demonstrated the ways kinship could be lethal.[14] Jaina inhabited the present in which a relationship could survive because of an imagined future, by preparing herself for the betrayals that were projected to take place in the future. Shamsheri, on the other hand, felt the betrayal in the present deeply and imagined vengeance in the future.[15]

Inhabiting these temporal projections results from the change in the status of brothers after becoming householders and the consequences this had for the relationship between siblings. An example of this change could be seen in the story Jaina told me about caring for her sister Jaira Bibi's family. Jaira was widowed very early in her youth and was left with four children, two sons and two daughters. Her husband's family was poor and had not been able to help her at all; she had had to move out of her husband's home and return to her natal home. Jaina had taken over responsibility for Jaira's care and raised all four children and in turn earned all their affection and love. In addition to getting the boys apprenticed with the ironmonger (who had been her lover in her youth), she organized the daughters' marriages. She told me, "I went to my three brothers and said, 'Look, you walk with your families, I don't. If you can give me some money for the marriage then that is okay, but I won't force you.' They gave me some money but I had to raise most of the money myself." She sold bits and pieces of her land to raise money for the marriages and was easily able to take out loans to make up the rest. Most of Jaina's life and material resources had been spent in raising her sister's orphaned family. Jaina was extremely proud of the loyalty and goodwill she had garnered by the work she had done for Jaira's family. She would often tell me the story of how one day she had fallen ill and fainted, and when she came about, she found Jaira's family gathered around her bed, worried, weeping.

Jaina knew that her brothers would not help their widowed sister Jaira get her daughters married. They would not give Jaira enough money, and she would understand and excuse her brothers' betrayal by saying that their primary responsibility was to their wives and their own children, not to their widowed sister. Jaina's taking care of the widowed sister and children was a form of participation in the family drama that shifted the stakes in maintaining kin ties because Jaina had no direct stakes in their lineage or thus the future it promises; they do not carry her name. Jaina would teach me irately about the ways of the world when I would ask her why she didn't live permanently with Jaira's family, since they clearly loved her so much: "You don't have a brain, will they see to their own family or to me? They have wives and children to take care of now [*Kuch aql nahin hai—unlog apne parivar ke saath chalenge ki mujhe dekhenge-unka family ho gaya hai, family ka dekhbhaal karna hoga*]."

The betrayals of which Jaina spoke are the inevitable betrayals that result from brothers becoming householders; hijras' critique of this form of kinship comes in the form of Jaina helping her widowed sister. But Jaina could only help Jaira because she did not have a household of her own. It is this form of relating that prevents kinship from becoming bestial, I argue, or prevents kin relations from becoming relations between animals, by reconfiguring circumstances that would have rendered brothers and sisters burdens that are resented, making betrayal inevitable.

THE *MAHABHARATA* OF THIS WORLD

Let me offer another ethnographic case to clarify what I mean. Mehraj lived in a one-room hut made of mud and straw, its entire back wall precariously tilting outward. Mehraj often tried to grow some vegetables in the patch of land next to her hut, a huge garbage dump, but the floods frequently ruined her crops, their viability already threatened by the putrid runoff from the garbage heap. For the most part Mehraj lived on alms from begging near the mosque or from *zakat* (obligatory charity) during the holy month of *Ramzan*. Her lovers at a nearby eatery took care of her and let her do odd jobs like waitressing or washing dishes and giving food or money in return. She had a bull calf whose balls she would often grab, making sex noises and asking the animal whether he would fuck her. Mehraj was also having a rough time because the community-based organization (CBO) believed that she had a lot of money saved in a bank account. Akhtari had once seen Mehraj's bank passbook and spread the rumor that she had thousands of rupees. Mehraj asked me, "If I had so much money would I be living like this—without any clothes or slippers, with a broken wall and door, and no food? The money that Akhtari saw, my mother collected from her children [Mehraj's brothers] and gave it to me for safekeeping. How can I spend it? What if she asks for it? She is an old woman, she will need it for her funeral; if I spend it, what will I give her then?" At that moment a girl from the neighborhood came and asked Mehraj why she hadn't eaten. Mehraj screamed and asked, "Who will prepare, cook, and take on these hassles of the world [*Kaun banayega, pakayega, duniya ka mahabharat*]?" Every interview with Mehraj over the last five years had in some way focused on her toothache. Because she would not brush her teeth, she was losing them and was in constant pain. I would take her to the doctor every year, and the doctor would prescribe medicines, which we would later buy, but Mehraj would inevitably stop gargling or taking the medicines after a week, saying, "I don't like it." She would irritably spurn any suggestion of taking medicines by saying, "Who will bother with the *mahabharata* of the world?"

It is the ubiquity of such mundane references to the *Mahabharata* that makes me turn to it. While philosophers and Indologists have seen it as a canonical text, there is a certain vocabulary that it secretes that seeps into the everyday. *Mahabharata*, the great epic of fratricidal violence, would often be used to index the family drama in rural Odisha. Mehraj used the word to signal how irritated she was with the world or to signify any bother that one has to undertake to live in this world—from cooking to taking medications to going out for errands, fixing her house, or working. Her experience of time was not marked with anxieties toward her own future but rather toward her mother's funeral. Putting herself on a temporal arc that focused on her mother's death and not on her own transformed Mehraj's present in ways I shall discuss further.

Mehraj was the only person whom all the hijras said had the right to beg because—unlike Akhtari, who had three sons-in-law to support her— Mehraj did not have any relatives. Mehraj had never held a job in her life but lived by begging and what can only very vaguely be called prostitution, because Mehraj would never solicit customers, nor would she ask them for money. Men would slip into her hut at night, and some of them would sometimes give her some money. I asked her why she didn't ask for money from all of them, and she said, "Who will bother asking them? They won't even give ten rupees if they don't want to." Her ten chickens were not big enough to lay eggs, and neither were her five ducks. Her lovers were usually rickshaw pullers or workers at the small *dhaaba* (roadside eatery). I use the term "lovers" instead of "customers" because not only were they not anonymous, but their relationships went beyond monetary or sexual transactions. I imagined these men cared for her because they would allow her to work erratically at the small eatery and take some dinner in return. None of Mehraj's neighbors, lovers, or other hijras expected that she would ever return the money she borrowed because they knew she had neither a family nor a job, and she was now too old to join a traditional *hijra gharana*. I discovered later that Mehraj did have family, but she would never go visit any of them. They came once or twice a year with some food for her, but that was the extent of their interaction. When I asked why she didn't go visit them, she would lament, "I don't like all this, I want to stay away from the *mahabharata* of this world." The word referring to the epic in these allusions might be seen in some instances as a metonymy for the world, in others as an allegory for everything that happens in this world.

When I asked Mehraj why she could not sell the chickens and ducks, she said they were not big enough. As Mehraj did not have money to buy feed, she collected garbage from the eatery where she ate—composed mainly of used tea leaves and vegetable peels—and mixed it with water to feed her animals. This rendered the animals undernourished and unhealthy, and, as happened in previous years I had known her, the animals died before becoming marketable. Since Mehraj expected them to die, yet hoped they would remain alive, the way she treated them was interesting, often cursing them because of their constant hungry clucking and quacking but then feeling worried if she could not find them.

I want to highlight the pedagogical import of this scene. A lot of young hijras were treated quite brutally by their family members. I remember Pawan hijra looking subdued and then noticed that she was covered in bruises. I asked Damru what the matter was, and she told me that Pawan hijra's family members must have beaten her up. When I asked why, Damru said, "Till you bring money into the house you have no value (*keemat*); they will keep on beating you. They used to beat me up, they used to beat Gungi. When I started earning and Gungi started doing *dhandha* (sex work), then they were very nice. Pawan hijra does not have a job—who will pay to have sex with her, she is so ugly? In fact, she has to give money to them to sleep with her." The animals that Mehraj kept had no value either—like children who did not earn, they were unhealthy, would die every year, and she had a bull instead of a cow with milk—yet she took care of them, irritated by their clucking, but concerned nonetheless. I will rely on the concept of animality and its reflection on kinship through the remainder of the chapter to argue that Mehraj and her animals evoke a way of negotiating kinship that prevents it from becoming bestial.

I have framed Mehraj's relationship with her animals as one of kinship to highlight the analogy that I am drawing between being animal and being kin. While there are other ways of talking in ordinary language about being related, there is a certain perdurability of the figure of the animal in analogies and metaphors when describing the corrosion of familial relations. This perduring symbology makes me want to open up the theme of the animal even if I am unable to bring it to a satisfactory resolution or conclusion. I will discuss some of the relevant material later in this and the following chapter. For now, I want to rely on the allegory of familial intimacy articulated through the animal as one that illuminates a certain disappointment that hijras felt in their kin relations.

YANNEHASTI NA TADKVACIT:
WHAT IS NOT HERE IS NOWHERE ELSE

It is said of the *Mahabharata*, the great epic of fratricide, that "what is not here is nowhere else." Unsurprisingly, then, this is where I begin to trace the relationship between hijras and their brothers. A. K. Ramanujan wrote, "Not *dharma*, the good life of right conduct, but *dharmasuksmata* or the subtle nature of *dharma* that mixes good and evil in every act, the impossible labyrinth of the moral life, is the central theme of the *Mahabharata*. So, the character of every person and the propriety of every major act is the subject of endless debate and moral scrutiny."[16] I have already noted that Jaina's awareness of her brothers' refusal to help the widowed sister in order to look after their own families is an awareness of the inevitable betrayal of intimacy. The morality of this betrayal, in the light of Ramanujan's words, cannot be pinned down very easily because it is an act that arises out of the split between the individual's duties as a householder and as a brother.

Veena Das comments on fraternal conflict in her seminal essay on Punjabi kinship: "Brothers who are fighting over property are described as dogs fighting over a bone. The term *sharika*, which may be translated as male agnates, or co-parceners, implies conflict. . . . Thus hostility between brothers, though expected and to an extent natural, is considered less than human. It implies that greed over property has made them relinquish even the biological ties established by their having shared the same womb and sucked the same milk. This hostility can never be legitimized, either in terms of human values or in terms of moral values of honor and face."[17] Although I agree with Das that fratricide can never be legitimized on any terms, I would argue that land or property inflects this hostility and squabbling between brothers precisely in terms of honor and face, in terms of dharma, thereby legitimizing fratricide in the inescapable terms she outlines—as "natural," "expected," but "less than human." What Jaina interprets as brothers forsaking their siblings to look after their own sons and daughters, and what Shamsheri refers to as the moral relationship between fathers and sons, I am understanding here in terms of dharma. Fratricide may not be legitimized, but violence between brothers is also a violence between fathers who need to secure inheritances for their own sons. The householder's concerns and loyalties shift when his intimacies include his wife and children, and this shift might have painful repercussions for his siblings and parents. But this is expected and is not treated so much as immoral as the inevitable corruption of relationships that time brings about. This is what Jaina meant when she said that her brothers will have to walk with their families, look after them into the future, rather than look behind after Jaina or their widowed sister.

I am forced to rely on dharma to complicate Das's analysis of fratricide because the word was used by Shamsheri to make me understand where exactly her grievances lay. The relationship that Jaina, Shamsheri, and Mehraj have with their families makes much more sense when we view the family drama through the lens of the *Mahabharata*. To illuminate how certain intimacies may require us to become bestial, let us consider how the figure of the dog as it appears in Hindu cosmology might legitimate behaving like a dog. Emily Hudson recounts a famous moment in the *Mahabharata*: "As Yudhisthira proceeds with the dog, Indra appears, inviting him to enter heaven in his human form. . . . Yudhisthira requests that the dog be allowed to accompany him, but Indra refuses. Yudhisthira insists. Then, as if by magic, the dog is transformed into the god Dharma, who tells Yudhisthira that he disguised himself in order to test Yudhisthira."[18] The fact that dharma—here in the role of death—can take the form of a dog implies that certain intimacies are death-dealing.[19] Land is the indispensable medium for that fight, but this is less a consequence of its economic value than the strong affective value it carries in this world.

Exemplifying this, an article published by the BBC entitled, "India Bihar Families Fight for Sixty-Six Years over a Plot of Land" reports that two families in Bihar had fought continuously over a plot of land for more than four generations and were preparing the fifth to carry the baton. As the land has been inundated and "turned into a riverbed," it is now worth only fifteen thousand rupees, hardly enough to compensate the two million rupees that one of the families had spent on the litigation. Even when the court ruled in favor of one family, the case was not settled, and appeals were filed by the other. One litigant in the reportage explains this form of self-destruction: "Now, it is more a battle for honor and prestige than for a piece of land."[20]

The epic fight between the Kauravas and the Pandavas and the competing claims between the two sets of patrilateral cousins have been well studied. Here I wish to focus on one moment before the battle of Kurukshetra to illustrate the relevance of land to fratricide that is the condition of kinship. The episode occurs after the Pandavas come back from their exile. The kingdom has been divided between the two sets of cousins, but as Matilal notes, it did not produce an overall good result: "The hostility between the Kauravas and the Pandavas started with redoubled force when the Pandavas became both prosperous and popular enough to arouse envy in the mind of Duryodhana."[21] After the period of their exile was over, the Pandavas demanded the return of their half of the kingdom. They were told by Sanjaya (who had been granted divine vision, thus could see the future) that "if the Kurus will not grant you your share, Ajata-shatru [literally, "one who had vanquished all his enemies"] without resorting to war, then in my opinion, a life of begging in the kingdom of the Andhaka Vrishnis would be better than winning your kingdom through war."[22] The Pandavas refuse to give up their plans to go to war but offer a compromise, saying that they would patiently bear all the insults that had been heaped upon them, if they were given five villages: "Give a single region of your kingdom to us, for we want peace: Avisthala, Vrikasthala, Makandi, Varanavrata, and let some boundary area be the fifth part. Give five villages to five brothers, Suyodhana."[23] Duryodhana, hearing of this request, assumed that the eldest of the Pandavas, Yudhishthira, was settling for such a small share of land "because he is afraid of [Duryodhana's] army and power."[24] Not even five villages from the powerful kingdom were parted with to be given to the Pandavas. Vidur says to him, "The Pandavas want to take just five villages, my lord, but you have no intention of giving them to them—you will not make peace."[25]

Dhritarashtra, the blind king who is Duryodhana's father and the Pandavas' paternal uncle, is emblematic of what I want to highlight about kinship; he is not willing to go against his son and forbid his going to war, nor is he willing to broker peace by giving up five villages, let alone half his kingdom. He will certainly not give up the entire kingdom, which belongs to his nephews according to some arguable rules. His anger is directed at himself for his inability to turn away from war and fratricide (and toward his son for not compromising) when only he, as the king, can put an end to the conflict by dividing the kingdom. His son obviously sees no reason to give up even five villages. Land is not the issue over which the brothers are fighting. If it were, then five villages would have been given to the Pandavas. Peace, though desired, is rendered unattainable because the Pandavas will not live under Duryodhana, but land is the necessary substrate over which the great drama can take place. Thus, while property and kinship obviously are related, the relationship is not causal; rather, property renders visible what is hidden in kinship.

Whereas the epic battle of Kurukshetra evokes an instance of fratricide that is the condition of kinship, in Bhadrak, the battle raged because of the brother's transformation into a householder. Veena Das comments on simmering hostilities between a householder's wife and her husband's family, which often brings the householder to choose between his loyalties to his wife (sexuality) and to his mother/brother/father/sister (kinship). Das's informant shows remorse after slapping his brother "for a mere woman" by saying that he was going to kill himself, and when prevented from doing so, that he would "cut off his own hand with which he had slapped his brother"—thus assuaging hostilities between the brothers. "In the context of the joint family," Das writes, "the rules of kinship morality stress the disguising of ties generated by shared sexuality, as well as ties generated by procreation."[26] We can read Shamsheri's brother's betrayal in a similar vein. We see that Shamsheri was not upset about the fact that her brother had used her to gain a second wife—his sexuality was understandable—but about the fact that he did not come see her in jail even to feign contrition, let alone express actual regret. This was the betrayal that was deeply felt by Shamsheri and that she was going to redress through robbing him of his land. The divided loyalties of the householder to his biological family, on the one hand, and his procreated family, on the other, bring into relief the temporal frames by which he is divided, as well. One frame involves circulation of money and medicine that he can offer to help support his siblings; the other involves circulation of inheritances and bequeathals of land that he has to offer his children. This is a dialectic of kinship and sexuality, or of fraternal amity and sexual affinity, each undoing but also fertilizing the ground for the other.

Jaina often made fun of Shamsheri's morose lamentations. She would ask her to laugh and joke, to inhabit the present, by forgiving her brother rather than plotting to exact revenge. Jaina was not asking Shamsheri to give up the fight because she was going to lose it anyway, but rather to walk away from it, in Mehraj's words, to "stay away from the *mahabharata* of this world." Though Jaina often claimed that she could sell her land if she needed the money, in fact, she never did sell the land. There were sporadic attempts, furtive whisperings between Jaina and several men who wanted to buy her land, but no deal ever went through. Jaina, even if she wanted to, could not sell her land because, as she pointed out, she might be murdered by her brothers for doing so. Shamsheri, even if she won the fight with her brother and gained possession of the land, would not have anybody to whom she could bequeath it, and her brother's family would eventually reclaim it. Jaina was asking Shamsheri to wake up to this reality and not be reduced to fighting like a dog over a bone. If householders become bestial toward each other over property and, in Das's words, forget the kinship they have with their mothers because of the sexuality they share with their wives, then hijras offered us a glimpse of what it would mean not to become bestial, not to forget kinship, and to stay away from the *mahabharata* of this world. In what follows, I argue that this staying away and remembering to be human, not turning bestial, is an exercise in restraint and a form of doing kinship that hijras taught.

SOLD BY FATE

Lawrence Cohen plots the various cultural idioms that are used to render the body aged and the movement of the father from the powerful position as a head of the family to the space of dying. He writes in his work *No Aging in India,* "Two transitions marked the shifts in the perception of the old person's voice and weakness: *the loss of authority* and *the loss of usefulness.* Both were gradual and contested processes, but each marked, fitfully, a shift in how an old parent was heard. . . . The loss of usefulness, that is, of any significant interpersonal role within the household, was associated with emerging criticisms of the old person babbling meaninglessly (*bakbak, pat pat, barbar*)."[27] Here Cohen presents the tragedy that awaits the householders; meanwhile hijras, I argue, teach us a way of modulating that tragedy: Jaina by taking care of her widowed sister Jaira and her children; Shamsheri and Mangu (whom I shall discuss shortly), by taking care of their respective mothers, which prevented the family's descent into the Bad Family. Shamsheri's mother lived with her because none of her sons wanted to keep her. Shamsheri often lamented the fact that she did not have money for her mother's medicines and medical treatment yet would be seen dutifully taking care of her; the old blind woman, in turn, begged for food for herself and her hijra child, and that is how they would take care of each other. As already mentioned, when Jaina's sister returned as a young widow with four children, all below the age of seven, none of her brothers offered any support—only Jaina. Likewise, Mangu begged to make sure she could meet her bedridden mother's expenses.

By opting out of certain expectations of masculinity, hijras also opted out of the dialectic of biology and sexuality as it gets played out in kinship. The temporal ramification of this dialectic needs to be teased out. Since they were not going to become householders, their sexuality was never in contradistinction to their kinship. Quite the opposite, in fact: their opting out of procreation allowed them to participate in kinship in a way that prevented their mothers from becoming accusative voices pointing toward the bad family. Jaina knew very well that she could not participate in the temporality of property transmission, much as she held on to the possibility. She was trying to persuade Shamsheri that fratricidal impulse is only meaningful when there are sons for whom one can fight one's brothers. In staying away from the *mahabharata* of the world, she would save her life—losing it would hardly be a sacrifice, as there would be nobody to reap the rewards or even be witness.

Jaina's participation in the temporality of the everyday, and not necessarily in the temporality of property transmission, can be seen in other sites as well, such as in the relationships Jaina shared with her brothers' wives, who were quite demonstrative in their love for Jaina.[28] I wasn't aware of their secret transactions at the beginning of my fieldwork, but their beautiful relationships unfolded as I started to notice a certain recurrent conversation that would take place furtively, without speech, in front of everybody's eyes. Jaina, the child Muneeza, and I would lunch together in her room, in between the times the men and women lunched. Once I remarked that there was an unnecessary abundance of food placed before Jaina, Muneeza, and me, to which Jaina replied that both her *bahus* (sisters-in-law) insisted on giving her food from their kitchens: "If I eat from one kitchen, the other one will feel bad, so I told them both to give me food every day and for every meal, so that they don't fight and don't think I love one more than the other."

While we were supposed to be napping, the women would often come surreptitiously to the window and slip some money ranging from 50 to 300 rupees, never more, into Jaina's hand. They hardly ever said anything because Jaina, who seemed to be dozing, would be quite alert to the movements outside her window. If she had dozed off, they would whisper, "*Bade Bhaiyya*," and Jaina would get up. If people of the neighborhood were nearby, they would come to the window, pretend to rest their hands on the windowsill, and slip the money into Jaina's hand while loudly scolding Jaina to distract the onlookers: "*Bade Bhaiya*, why are you spoiling my children, you give them money to buy rubbish to eat from the market and now they won't eat rice properly." Nobody would suspect that behind these visits, ostensibly meant to chide Jaina gently for her avuncular indulgences, the women of the house were betraying their husbands.

The loud scolding would awaken me from my siesta, and, after a few weeks, my curiosity piqued, I too like Jaina began to pretend to be asleep and poked my head up whenever the transactions occurred, much to Jaina's mild irritation and amusement. Once I figured out what exactly was being slipped into her hand and hidden in tins in her cupboard, I goaded Jaina into telling me what was going on. With an exhausted sigh, she finally relented and let me in on the secret. The sisters-in-law would often save money from their household expenses, or earn it from odd jobs they would do, like filling rolled *bidis* (unfiltered cigarettes) with tobacco, or receive small amounts for the children from relatives during their visits, or money from various friends and relatives (including me) during the festival of Eid. They would give it to Jaina to deposit in a post office savings account for them. I asked Jaina why they did this and why it was so important that their husbands not catch wind of it. She replied:

> Because they love me and trust me, they know I won't tell their husbands, they come running, saying "Bade Bhaiyaa, please deposit this money for our children." If the husbands come to know they will take it away, they might also beat them up and say, "when I am here, what is the need to do all this, do we not take care of you and your children that you have to save money, do you not have any faith/trust [*bharosa*] in us." My father was also like that; once, when I was very young, eleven or twelve, we needed a lot of money. My mother told me to go sell her heavy silver armbands. My father, when he discovered this, beat her up very badly, screaming at her, "everybody will now know, they will taunt me that I can't run my own house." That's why I go and deposit the money in their accounts secretly.

The relationship between husbands and wives described here is not one in which legalistic definitions of cruelty or domestic violence have any bearing—there was without a doubt a lot of love between the married couples. But a structural tension and currency of distrust that travel a specific constellation of intimacy were also present. Das has written lucidly about the relationship that a woman's natal family continues to maintain with her even after her marriage. They inquire about her conjugal house and worry about the sexual adequacy of her husband and whether the young woman looks unhappy; members of the family with whom a joking relationship is shared can use their privileged familiarity to find out what troubles the young bride.[29]

Jaina, on the other hand, prescribed a very strict etiquette for the woman if she was unhappy in her marriage, while Das remarks that "parents, for all their advice to the daughters to consider the conjugal house as their own, would consider it unnatural if the daughter followed that advice to the letter, especially in the early years of marriage."[30] Jaina said:

> If a woman gets married and her husband doesn't touch her and he has told her on the first night of the marriage, "I did not have the heart to get married and my elders got me married forcefully, I don't have anything. *This*—my honor is now in your hands. If the wife now has pride, honor, and if she has knowledge (*ilm*), qualities (*sifat*), she will keep every-

thing to herself—this is very personal and delicate talk between a husband and a wife. After a few months of marriage, the woman has to go to her grandmothers. They will ask her and enquire whether she is okay, whether she has been impregnated or not. If they see she is sad they will enquire and she can either say, "I have not come to your house in mourning, so then you tell me—why else would I be so sad." They will understand immediately that the husband has not touched her and she has not felt the pleasures of a married woman. They will then see what needs to be done, whether she should get divorced; they will talk to the boy's family and everybody will know that the husband is not a man. But if she is an intelligent, honorable woman then she will tell them, "Listen, this is between my husband and me, why are you asking me all this?" She will tell them, "Everything is okay." After a few years, she will obviously not have become pregnant, and people will still enquire. She should then say, "Everything is fine between my husband and me but if I don't have children in my destiny (*naseeb*), then what can I do?" Then that woman has no other choice but to hope that death comes to her quickly in a few years. The husband must then realize: "If my wife had opened her mouth, I would have been insulted and humiliated, people would call me a hijra, a maichiya, but she kept her mouth shut. She had knowledge, good qualities, she hid everything about me." So now, he has to give her respect, he has to go to her grave often and offer a new shroud, garlands of flowers, incense, because he has to be grateful that his wife kept everything within herself and protected him.

This edict issued to the woman to quietly suffer explains the relationship Jaina had with sisters-in-law. She was aware that they might be suffering quietly, resigned to their fate, and to make their lives bearable she colluded with them in betraying their husbands.

Das, in her essay "Kama in the Scheme of Purusharthas: The Story of Rama," writes that Sita had to renounce her life to irrevocably establish the legitimacy of her sons and consequently restore the lineage of her husband.[31] Jaina metes out an equally harsh prescription for the daughter-in-law who has to wait patiently for death if married to a husband who cannot sexually satisfy her; she should invoke God and her cruel fate as excuses to explain her childlessness to others to save the honor of her husband. Given such rules, the tensions arising from suspicion and accusation toward daughters-in-law can be enough to drive them to death, as has been recorded and studied by generations of scholars, writers, and thinkers.[32] Jaina's collusion with her daughters-in-law attenuated these tensions—tensions that even goddesses have not survived—through secrecy and solidarity. Jaina displaced and repositioned the betrayal away from the fight over land inheritance into the everyday realm. These betrayals, I argue, not only help to sustain the lineage—the women were saving money to spend it on the children who bore their husband's name—but also help to sustain the family in everyday domestic existence.

The Hindu god Ram himself could not protect his lineage from being maligned as polluted and was required to renounce Sita. Jaina's brothers were only mortal, and in the local moral world of Bhadrak even little gestures, such as their wives hiding money secretly earned, would have been sufficient cause for them to be denigrated as incompetent and unmanly. The relationship between Jaina and her sisters-in-law, and her widowed sister's family, and the relationship Shamsheri, Mangu, Mehraj, and many other hijras in Bhadrak had with their mothers, brokered the domestic space in their brothers' households. Hijras ask us to reexamine the self-sufficiency of heteronormative reproduction at least in the conditions of poverty. They press the irony that though the family may be created through the relationships between father, mother, and children, the domestic sphere requires a host of other characters to pacify the mood of the house and render it livable or to preserve it from destroying itself.[33]

A hijra's position, though, makes her vulnerable to fraternal violence when seen through the logic of alliance. Given that she does not marry or produce children, she refashions the protocols of intimacy to make a place for herself in the domestic sphere, if not the family, and instructs in practicing kinship, adhering to "laws," which may not be legal in any formal sense. For example, the relationship between what was a male body (the hijra's) and her sister-in-law's became one not of leviratic possibility but one of friendship. In punctuating the transformation of a son into a householder who usurps authority from his father and betrays his mother "for a mere woman," hijras also stay away from the *mahabharata* of the world in a way that allows them not to become dogs but instead to remain human and take care of old parents. The renunciation of hijras might at first glance seem to place them in opposition to the family, but their participation in kinship via mothers, sisters, and sisters-in-law helps to sustain certain family relations. I read these ways of participating in the family as a diagonal entrance, one that does not create or destroy but preserves families and hence lineages. The difference and distance between creating and preserving, on the one hand, versus preserving and destroying, on the other, are the difference and distance between value and price—a dead sister-in-law and a live one.

FAMILIES WE FUCK

Lest I be accused of fetishizing the relationship between hijras and their mothers and other women of their family, I must offer another scene exemplifying how kinship can be redone. Tappi lived in Gabasahi, which is a small settlement between the town of Bhadrak and Charampa train station, on a large piece of land worth Rs.32 lakhs [3,200,000 INR / 60,000 USD] that formerly belonged to her grandfather and was now divided between her father, paternal uncle, and paternal aunt. The father's piece of land had three small rooms under one hut; one room was occupied by Tappi, and the other two were rented out (for 325 and 350 rupees) to three men from Dhamnagar who would come to Bhadrak to sell their wares at the train station. Tappi lived on the rent collected from the tenants. The land also had an outhouse and a tube well that she shared with her uncle, who lived in another more solidly built house of bricks next to her hut. The unmarried, constantly inebriated uncle and Tappi's grandmother lived together with Tappi's male cousin (FZS).[34] There was a lawsuit pending between Tappi's father and his sister, Tappi's aunt, regarding the division of land; in fact, the aunt lived directly behind Tappi's plot, and they shared a border. Her father had a railway job at Paradeep, a neighboring district, where he lived with his wife, Tappi's mother, and their other son; he rarely came to Gabasahi. Tappi's mother often asked her elder son and his cousins to beat up Tappi because she was roaming around wearing saris, bangles, and makeup. To escape her family, Tappi had run away to Gujarat and Rajasthan, where she worked at a thread factory in 2006; she had returned to Gabasahi in 2009—when I made her acquaintance—not to her mother's but to her aunt's house, which was behind her present location. Her father had built these three rooms after the supercyclone of 2005, which had destroyed almost everything in that area because of the floods. Tappi told me that her father was very fond of her, but since (she added a bit irritatedly) her mother controlled the purse strings in the house, her father could not do anything in front of her mother. Tappi's mother often told her that because Tappi earned money by fucking around (*dhanda karke*), there was no need for her to ask for money from home—that is, to take the rent that was collected from the tenants. Once she even threatened to kick Tappi out of her room and give that up for rent as well.

Her mother often came to Bhadrak with her elder son, threatening to put an end to Tappi's way of living, and Tappi's friends and allies got used to receiving panicked phone calls asking for help because she feared she was going to be beaten up by them. I too began receiving phone calls asking for help, but Jaina stopped me from going by saying, "This is her daily problem, nothing will happen, don't worry." When I looked unconvinced, she said, "I live here, I know everything; if you go you will also get beaten up. Don't worry, smoke a cigarette, drink your tea, Tappi has plenty of men to help her. She will raise one finger and ten men will jump up to save her." I acquiesced, and the next day when I met Tappi she didn't look any worse for wear. I asked her what had happened the day before. She replied:

> [My mother] doesn't live here, so people don't know her and her son. If they beat me up, all the men here who know me will come to save me. Remember the last time you came and you saw my aunt's son and asked me what had happened to him—because he was so hurt and wounded he couldn't even walk? I said it was nothing, my mother and my brother came to kick me out, they started beating me, I screamed loudly and all my men [*chahne waale*] came and thrashed the three of them. Since then, they come and threaten, but they will not touch me. They have learned their lesson, and I have no problems. Come, say whatever you want to say, I won't be here to listen; I see them, I run away.

No one took Tappi's panicked calls seriously because they knew there would be plenty of people there to save her, not least because she had slept with most of them, but also because her tenants/lovers were three muscular men who were very fond of her. Her house would have a constant stream of visitors dropping by; in fact, during all my interviews the place had people coming and going to smoke ganja, drink, or have sex. She would also charge exorbitantly for sex—600 rupees for a fuck—but only from men she did not know who came from areas she was unfamiliar with. When asked why, she said, "The men here already do so much for me, I can't charge them, they are brothers/friends (*bhailog*). But outsiders, I will charge them, and I won't do it anywhere but a lodge."

Kath Weston, in her groundbreaking ethnography on gay kinship, observes, "When lesbians and gay men in the [San Francisco] Bay Area applied kinship terminology to their chosen families, they usually placed themselves in the relationship of sisters and brothers to one another, regardless of their respective ages."[35] To this I would add—in Tappi's case—that, regardless of rules of incest as well, she called all the men with whom she undertook transactions of care *bhaiyya*, or "elder brother." I am aware that this word is a common way of addressing the entire world of South Asia, but the men milling around Tappi would often tell me, "We are like her elder brothers. She cooks for us when we come to Bhadrak, she takes care of us, so why wouldn't we take care of her?" One of these men, who at that time was her most important lover, told me, "I can give my life for her as well. Brothers are always ready to sacrifice their lives for their sisters." As Weston pointed out, the families that lesbians and gay men choose usually do not have intergenerational relationships but fraternal and congenial ones: they are brothers and sisters, friends and lovers.

The antagonism between Tappi and certain members of her family arose from the fact that Tappi was a hijra. Once again it played out for her as it commonly did through land property. Her mother's demands that she stop fucking around, wearing makeup and saris, behaving like a hijra were inextricably bound up with her demand that Tappi stop taking the rent from the tenants and give up occupying one of the rooms. However, Tappi participated in the *mahabharata* of the world and wrested control of the land— yet she has no one to whom to bequeath it. The Pandavas, who won the epic war in the *Mahabharata*, faced a similar situation: all their kin had died in the war, leaving an heirless state that was only resolved by Krishna reviving a dead baby that would allow the world to continue.[36] The dispute between Tappi and her family would be resolved in the future with Tappi's death and her brother's children inheriting the land, I felt sure, but for the time being she had her land, and she defended her right to it with the support and protection of her lover-brothers.

Tappi can be seen as participating in the *mahabharata* of the world, in the fratricidal war over land—but not because of land. Lacking anyone to bequeath her land pushes our analysis of kinship and land toward questions of temporality. How do brothers sustain tenderness and arrest time, whose inexorable march demands that brothers betray each other to become fathers and look to the future? In Tappi's peculiar case we have a strange country where the logic of kinship dilates to calculate everybody as brothers; here there are no fathers or sons between whom the land is entrusted. With that dilation the rules of incest are collapsed, with lovers becoming brothers.[37] This becomes a mimetic reflection of segmentary affiliation, wherein it is not a question of brothers who shared a womb united against the world, but of unrelated men—strangers becoming brothers—fighting against the brothers who are related by blood.

THIS IS HOW THE LAND LIES

Until now my argument has been that hijras, by living with their families, experience kinship in two different temporal orders. The first is instantiated in the present by the attentiveness offered by their brothers in the everyday circulation of food, money, and medicines; the second is the imagined future transmission of property. In sidestepping the order of reproduction and pro-creation, hijras are wary of participating in the fratricidal war that inevita-bly takes place in the form of contestation over land—inevitably, because brothers become householders in order to agonizingly reproduce the social. Walking away from becoming householders allows hijras to walk away from participating in this fraternal war. The shift in temporal orders from futu-rity to the present, I have shown, may allow them to take care of their mothers, preventing the latter's voices from becoming *barbar* and their fam-ilies from becoming the "bad family." In the case of Jaina, walking away from participating in lineage—but not from the family, the household, the domestic—allowed her to prevent her widowed sister from becoming a bur-den. Furthermore, Mehraj, Mangu, and Jaina, instead of betraying their brothers for land, would collude in betraying their brothers for more peace-able ends: Mehraj and Mangu, by saving up for their mother's funeral away from the prying eyes of their siblings, whose responsibility it should have been in the first place; and Jaina, by conspiring with her sisters-in-law to render the mood of the household more salubrious.

Leo Bersani, in his article "Father Knows Best," offers a provocative read-ing of Claire Denis's film *Beau Travail*, about a group of legionnaires posted in Djibouti. Bersani interprets the film as a "family story": he elaborates the inexplicable antagonism between the master sergeant, Galoup, and the beau-tiful legionnaire, Sentain, as indicative of a "fratricidal impulse" that is con-solidated by the "fraternal bond," which the legion and Forestier, the father figure in the film, constantly signal. Bersani focuses his interpretation on the last scene and specifically the last shot of the film. He writes, "Stand up and simply leave the family tragedy by which Western culture has been oppressed at least since Oedipus's parricide.... Leave the violence of a desire for the father and the son, a violence that transforms brotherhood into fratricide."[38] I would like to propose that hijras can be seen as walking away from the family drama and the future promised by becoming a householder; but unlike the master sergeant, they do not do so after an agonizing education in the violence and criminality that found the family. Because they are more than aware that brothers kill each other, while they remain with their families they "modulate its obscene destructiveness" by participating in it in ways that adhere to a logic of sustenance. Betrayals of their brothers in the present help to prevent betrayals in the future, and, as a consequence, the brothers of hijras are less prone to fight like dogs over the land.

Thus, hijras, when fucking in the fields, offered lovers a respite from being human, and meanwhile in their household they offered respite to their brothers, forfending their becoming animals—fighting like dogs—and reducing parental voices to abject meaningless sounds. Mehraj goes a step further and makes animals her kin: she cares for animals even though they are not, and do not become, economically viable. She shows concern when they are lost—as if they were kin—despite being irritated by their constant clucking to express a hunger that she cannot afford to assuage. Hijras take care of parents and punctuate the ceaseless pathological, even perverse, repetition of social reproduction of animals undertaken by householder brothers. Let me offer a few thoughts to clarify hijras' interventions, which might also be considered an inversion of the diktat of Indian cosmic theory that provides the paradigm for the tense battlefield that is the household.

Lawrence Cohen comments on a widely circulated folktale that allegorizes the transfiguration of a man from a son into a householder, and later into a family burden. He writes:

A man's aging is illustrated through a bestiary. Against the cosmic theories of *asramadharma* [there is] a refiguring of the life course in terms of three distinct but each unpleasant forms of dehumanization. Adulthood here peaks at forty, envisioned as the burden of carrying along one's wife and weak sons. Sixty remains the time of political inversion, when the meaning of debility shifts from the burden of the powerful (the father as ox) to the subordinate duties of the grandfather (the father as dog). After sixty, the voice becomes central, the abject request of the man forced to beg from his own son. At eighty, a different meaning of senility is offered, not the political abjection of the dog, but the far more embodied decay of the voiceless old man, for whom the request has degenerated thoroughly into meaninglessness: the monkey.[39]

The tragic narrative presented earlier is a gendered narrative. Cohen argues that for women, becoming dogs was a formal resistance to becoming like cows—regarded as holy, but a hassle nonetheless. Hijras, I have argued, by their participation in the family, prevented their mothers from becoming holy hassles and prevented their mothers' voices from signaling toward the bad family, senility, or abject dehumanization, while their brothers were prevented, at least in one account, from fighting like dogs. To understand the temporal implications of this humanity—and this humanization—I must begin by looking at the line in the *Bhagwat Purana* that reads, "One should treat animals such as deer, camels, asses, monkeys, mice, snakes, birds, and flies exactly like one's own son. How little difference there actually is between children and these innocent animals."[40] It is the way of the world in Bhadrak that children, who are like innocent animals, grow up to become householders who then subsequently treat the aging bodies of their parents like animals, and are eventually, when old, treated like animals themselves. In a different vocabulary, it could be said that in refusing to subscribe to this series of transfigurations and its temporality, hijras were subscribing to a different order of semiosis.[41] In taking care of their mothers and not fighting with their brothers over land, hijras established a different suturing of the present to the past and the future. Resisting the order of history that made parents into dogs and monkeys meant that the past did not become past, and in abstaining from fighting with their brothers, staying away from the *mahabharata* of this world, the future did not loom as the future. Instead, what remained was the present, and a republic in which all were human—and humanized—even the animals.

A LIFE WELL DIED

Let me recount another instance of how the past, present, and future were reconfigured, or sutured differently, to allow for a different temporality of semiosis, with different commitments and entitlements. Mangu's house stood on a plot of land that was formerly owned by her maternal grandmother, but now belonged to her mother. The household had seven members besides Mangu: her bedridden blind mother, her sister and brother-in-law, the brother-in-law's daughter (who had fled her husband's house after being beaten up by him), and this young woman's child, plus the two sons of another sister. Mangu had the responsibility of running the entire household. When I asked her why her nephews didn't contribute, she replied in an even tone, without resentment.

> M: No, they don't contribute at all. They eat here, sleep here, both of them have jobs, but they won't give me even one rupee.
> V: Well, you should kick them out then, why do you have to feed them?
> M: [calmly] No, that's not possible. When you came here two years ago, didn't you see how the house was falling? You had to duck low to enter, and when you straightened up too quickly you hurt yourself on the iron rod—do you remember how much your back bled?
> V: Yeah, I remember. [I removed my *kameez* to show her the scar.]
> M: Well, to fix the house they asked me for 60,000 rupees and they said, "If you don't give it then we will throw you out."
> V: But how can they do that?
> M: They can. They will say, "Oh, this is a hijra who doesn't give anything but just eats here; why should we let you stay here?"
> V: But they should share (*mil baat*) and live.
> M: That's what I tell them, but they don't listen. They don't care about their own nani. They will throw both of us out—they are young men—and then where will I go with my mother?

Mangu's position as a hijra made her vulnerable to being utilized in a particular way by her family members. Mangu was well aware that they could decide to kick her off the land where she was living and that she would not be able to handle the court expenses that the litigation would entail. This resulted in Mangu sustaining a household of seven others that lived off her earnings.[42] I suppose there is something to be said for supporting one's family and other animals—yet every time Mangu fell ill and was unable to go begging, her family would begin to complain about the expense of her medicines, the trips to hospital, the lack of food in the house, the demanding task of taking care of her. Mangu would then escape to a nearby *majhar* (the shrine of a Muslim saint) to stay until she recovered enough to resume earning.

Mangu once whispered to me that she had saved 10,000 rupees for her own funeral and another 10,000 for her mother's because she was sure that no one in the family would produce the funds needed to bury them properly. They would say, "Oh, this is a hijra, there is nobody of her own (*aage peeche koi nahin*) who will waste money on her funeral." Then she added, pleased as Punch, "Now, if I have money, why would I ask somebody to take care of me when I die? I will just say this is my money, please do this and this after my death. You need to do all this. Only if I have money can I carry my mother on my shoulders. Otherwise, what face will I show Allah, that I let my mother go alone to her grave?" Her faith in the world, and that her selfish family would use the money she gave them for the purposes of a proper funeral, puzzled me. Mangu would often talk with subdued excitement, imagining her funeral taking place; her eyes would light up and she would betray a slight, charming smile. The conversation would never seem morbid to either of us. She would begin, "You know, when I go, I want them to take out my corpse with a lot of celebrations, bathed and washed with expensive fresh flowers." Mangu's insistence on the beautiful funeral can be seen as her putting the final punctuation on the story of her life in which she had been rendered helpless by her family. Her funeral would render her the signatory of her life and would in effect legitimize her existence. The abject present would be impotent in the light of the splendid funeral, which would recast her life, these present moments, with new meaning. The meaning of her life was yet to come, and the betrayals of daily life would be erased. This is why, I suppose, in the evenings Mangu was at most stony-faced, never bitter or angry, with the demands of her greedy, parasitical family.

I met Mangu for the last time on August 6, 2013. She was once again at the *majhar*, doing very poorly. I had gone to her house to say good-bye, as I was leaving for Calcutta the next day; when I arrived, her sister began complaining before I even alighted from the motorbike. As soon I heard the word *majhar* in response to my inquiry as to Mangu's whereabouts, I zoomed away, leaving the shrieking harpy behind. At the *majhar*, Mangu spoke about how she was not feeling well, and now that her death was palpably near she did not make any mention of her funeral. I stared at her, wondering why a part of her neck was throbbing as if a bird were struggling to get out. We remained silent at the peaceful *majhar,* listening to the sounds of crickets, frogs, monkeys, dogs, cattle, distant motorbikes, and other sounds I could not make out. When dusk fell, I pressed some money in her hand and left (Jaina later assured me that the sister would snatch the money). Mangu died the next day. Jaina called me from the hospital to say that the sister was complaining about lack of money for a funeral. Upon inquiring, we learned that the family claimed that the money Mangu had saved had gone into treating her illness and taking care of the house—that they had no money—which no one believed because everyone knew that the nephews were working. Jaina was broke because she had given the sister 15,000 rupees for Mangu's expenses, and nothing remained of that, either. I offered to pay for the funeral, but Jaina told me it would be useless, since I wouldn't be there to supervise the spending, and they would just take the money and would not arrange a proper funeral. She said, "They will ask for ten thousand but they won't even spend two thousand." I asked her to oversee the funeral, but she said it would result in a fight because the sister would say, "Mangu is our family, just give us money and we will take care of it; you are an outsider." She continued, in an exhausted voice, "You don't understand, they are only after money—what kind of a world is this?" Finally, along with a lot of complaining about the expenses, Mangu was buried by her family without the funeral she wanted.

I began writing this account of Mangu five months before her death. I was going to offer her story as evidence of hijras negotiating relations with their families by inhabiting lifeworlds in which their abjection and helplessness would be erased in the event of a splendid funeral—a negotiation whereby the act is cleaved from accreting meaning immediately. The anthropologist Sophie Day remarks that sex workers in Britain organized their biographies in such a way that the past or the future appeared as a snapshot—an image, view, or resource that isolated the present and restricted "a disagreeable period in sex work to the short term, apart from the flow of life." She chose the term "snapshot" not only because it implies distance between the sex work of the present and the family of the past or future, but also because that distance brackets the present.[43] Mangu's funeral was, in her mind, if anything a snapshot—an image that allowed her to bracket the misery and exploitation that she faced at the hands of her extortive kin. If the funeral had been the grand ceremony she wanted, then it would have been a signature to her life and the ultimate revenge. It would have wrested her life back from the hands of her relatives, an abject existence in which she had been rendered helpless in her attempt to provide her mother a decent life and funeral. Nadia Seremetakis reminds us that a good death is marked by a good funeral, which further testifies to the good or ethical life led by the deceased person.[44] A good funeral for Mangu, similarly, would have prevented a reading of her life as abject. Did it fail or succeed, in the end? Although there were no expensive fresh flowers, or an expensive shroud, this snapshot of her future made Mangu's past and present more bearable; in the certitude of a beautiful funeral she negotiated relations with her family of spongers in an enviably unruffled manner. Perhaps it was success and failure simultaneously, a modulation partially abating the obscene destruction of the family that mortifies the flesh and renders one animal.

CONCLUSION: ROOMS AND RUINS

If one cannot address kinship through land or land through kinship, the loss that fraternal violence implies might be seen as melancholia. The loss of an object, the intimacy between brothers, results in a fight that takes form through the substratum of property but not because of it. By this I mean that brothers will inevitably participate in or make gestures toward forms of fratricide, or in other words, will fight like dogs once they have their own families and their loyalties are divided. Hijra occupy the place of a pedagogical figure: they betray in the present, rather than the future, and they do so to make the household livable. They turn away from becoming animal and ask their brothers to do the same; in this they adhere to laws that are not the laws of the land. The law of the land is that every householder becomes an animal at the hand of his sons, thus the battle the brother might have won is a preamble to the war that he will lose to his own children when he becomes an old man. To fight like dogs also means to become abject like the dog, then meaningless like the monkey, and finally nothing, when one's voice is not even heard. Hijras as pedagogical figures show that this becoming animal through adherence to kinship, which is the obscene destructiveness of the family, is not necessary and can be modulated, thus signaling toward the laws of preservation and sustenance.

Freud wrote in his iconic essay "Mourning and Melancholia" that "the patient is aware of the loss which has given rise to his melancholia, but only in the sense that he knows *whom* he has lost but not *what* he has lost in him."[45] All the hijras in Bhadrak and Bhawanipatna were aware that they would lose the affection and loyalties of their brothers because of the brothers' greed for land, and through that loss and greed they would also lose a certain form of intimacy. But the difference between the brothers and hijras is the difference between mourning and melancholia. The brothers had new objects to love and take care of; in fact, it was because of these new objects—in the form of wives and children—that this narrative of loss would take place. Hijras, on the other hand, did not. For hijras the loss remained as melancholia. This unapproachable quality of loss, coded again and again in the phrase "now they have wives and children, they will have to look to or walk with their own family," became available through ethnography.[46]

The brothers must have felt a loss as well, but not one that was unconscious. They were fighting, but this fighting like dogs was excused, rendered understandable, and even expected because they had to now walk with their own families. Hijras' loss was inevitably melancholic for them because there was no reason available to them that ratified this violence; in other words, they could not understand why kinship mortified the flesh in the way it did. But I want to argue that their participation in kinship was what Leo Bersani has called a "subversive passivity."[47] Hijras in Odisha, by remaining with their families and by participating in the institutions that reproduce the social, perhaps just repeat the violence that is inherent in the Oedipal drama. But this is a repetition that is different in that it punctuates progress: kin do not become animals, but animals become kin, all become brothers, and the funeral of the future robs the present of its sting. Let me offer a comparison of two sets of rooms and ruins to clarify my point.

One malevolent night in Bhawanipatna, all of us had returned from the hot spot where hijras solicit customers. We were all feeling irritated for some reason. We were getting on each other's nerves, and, very soon, squabbling broke out. We parted ways, and Nandita and I ended up with each other. We sat on the road, and she started speaking:

My parents didn't educate me so I could not study. Two friends of mine and I, when we were little, had to steal from the market stuff that we would later sell to get things for school—like a schoolbag, pencil box, and other things. Only if a child is given these things will he want to go to school, isn't it? I was not given anything and my parents were not strict with me so I started doing whatever I do. I won't lie to you, I used to steal a lot because my parents didn't give me anything. Once I asked my father to divide the land between us so that there would be no fighting between us, but my brothers who wanted my land came at me with a knife, saying they will kill me if I ask for my share. Only Dev [her nephew] protected me, and only because I had given him five thousand rupees for his tuition. I am not like Damru, I have no pride [*guroor*], I eat with what I earn [*main apna paisa ka khaati hoon*]. My eldest brother's wife has never slept with him, she has always slept with her Devar, my second brother. She stopped him from getting married, and when he wanted to get married and have children, I told him, "Listen get married, I will give you one lakh rupees," but she stopped him and said, "Are my children not your children?" Dev, Robin and their two brothers call him Bappa [they call their younger paternal uncle "father"]. Isn't that shameful? I would have left this place but what can I do, I have built this house, spent so much money; they will be happy to see me leave, but why should I? I have built this house. I had put in windowpanes, but my nephews broke them; they broke the sofa I bought, they broke everything—the cups and glasses, the windows and everything. They do nothing and are not even grateful that I give them food to eat every day. You have seen how they are always lounging about, sleeping in my bed all the time, watching my television. They are eyeing my money. Since there was this motorcycle accident, Dev is trying to get me to give him information about this account so that he can get the money, but I am scared he will run away with the money.[48] I can easily go to Jharsuguda to beg on the trains, but I don't want to leave my home behind; I have built it. Naina has asked me so many times to come to Jharsuguda to come beg with her, and she is very nice and I can do it.

After some talk about something else, she continued:

When I went to Jharsuguda—Naina only took me once with her—wouldn't you think that because she is my friend and brought me there, she would show me the ways to beg? She should have taken me with her. But after just one day she told me to go with some other hijra whom I didn't know. [Why did she do that? I asked.] Maybe because she would earn more money if she went alone and the thing is, they have sex on the trains, right? So she could not have sex in front of me because she is pretending to be *sati* [holier than thou] with me.

Nandita's house consisted of four rooms. Everybody slept there because one of her lovers in the neighborhood, an electrician, stole electricity for her from the nearby government transformer. The electricity meant that the television was always running, and, more importantly, there was an air cooler for hot summer nights. Since everybody was lounging there, fights also took place, resulting in the household things being mostly broken. She could only extract support from her nephews because she was feeding them three square meals a day and paying for their expenses such as travel, tuition, and clothes. She resented it but was helpless as to how she could consolidate her inheritance and her investments. The rooms she built were the only set built of bricks on the plot of land; the other two sets of rooms were in one hut and belonged to her two brothers. She wanted the land to be divided so that she could kick her family out, but nobody was going to help her do that.

The other set of rooms, which were in ruins, belonged to Bhawanipatna's most beautiful hijra, Damru, my primary informant in whose house I lived during my fieldwork. Damru herself was badgered all the time by her family regarding land matters. She and her mother lived in one of two rooms, which constituted half the hut. I lived in the other room. The other half was where her sister lived. Her sister had fallen in love with a Muslim man, and the man had been cast out from the community. The couple had shown up at Damru's door, and Damru had chosen to protect them. By the time I arrived they had a five-year-old kid. The neighborhood had revolted against this interfaith marriage by blocking the entrance to their house with a thatched wall; as a consequence, to enter their house one had to take a twenty-minute walk and enter from the back of the house, which was on the field where everybody went to shit. It was only when she got a tube well fixed in her courtyard that the neighborhood removed the wall, because it was a more convenient place to get water than from the government tube well down the road. Damru was more than aware of this bitter compromise.

The four rooms built beside the hut had no roofs, just bricks cemented into walls and partitions; there was no furniture, paint, or lime to smooth the walls, half-built and in ruins. Damru's mother would constantly ask her every morning to get them fixed and completed. When I asked her why she wasn't getting them fixed, she replied:

Look, once I get them fixed, my sister and brother-in-law will move here permanently. Now that the man and my sister have been accepted by his community because they have a child—nobody can fight their grandchild—they will sooner or later have to accept them. They are showing no signs of returning. Every week they say they will return but they are not returning. I know why. They want this land. Once I get these rooms fixed, they will move in there completely. My other sister, whose husband has left her for an old ugly prostitute, will also move in here. Then her husband will also return and they both will take over the land. What will I do? I am a hijra, no sons to take care of me or give my land to; they will kick me out. Now I have some land, they respect me, they need me, they need my money. But once they are here permanently, who will protect me? Don't they have money? Why can't they build it themselves?

Both the houses were in ruins, but while Nandita's ruins offer a narrative of violent kinship in that her hard work in building, painting, and making her house inhabitable was treated with carelessness by her nephews, Damru's ruins are anti-narrative. They were never completed or ever used and were already falling into disrepair. One of the rooms was used by everybody as a urinal and a trash dump—the past, present, and future of those ruins were not very discernible. Her family continued to live in their old thatched hut next to it, divided by a cupboard and a hastily put together wall. While both hijras were repeating the familial drama of fratricide, dispute over property, and loss of intimacies, Damru's ruins evoked Nandita's ruins, but with a promising difference.

Judith Butler brings Freud closer to the scene that I am seeking to analyze. She writes, "If in melancholia a loss is refused, it is not for that reason abolished. . . . If the object can no longer exist in the external world, it will then exist internally, and that internalization will be a way to disavow the loss, to keep it at bay, to stay or postpone the recognition and suffering of loss."[49] I want to read the negotiations that hijras set up with their families as this form of melancholia, which defers betrayal and the inevitable loss of land in the future. I suggest that Damru's refusal to complete building the rooms, like Jaina's betrayals, does repeat the narrative but with a difference that creates a temporal disturbance and domesticates the violence of the family.

Hijras' participation in their families is one version of the momentous possibility that Bersani discovers for us. The trash can within us, the fratricidal impulse, is inevitable for all of us, but there are ways to be non-cruel, ways to modify the obscene destructiveness of the family. Challenging the self-sufficiency of heteronormative reproductivity, hijras effectively divert a focus on "norms" as a site of power; they show that violence does not so much emerge from the violation of norm as being coded into kinship. Consequently, they destabilize notions of violation, transgression, and margin. Jaina calibrates her demands made on her brothers, while Damru defers the future when her sisters and brothers-in-law will kick her out of her house. Against Nandita's realization that there is betrayal in every intimacy, familial and nonfamilial, Mangu, Mehraj, and Tappi offer forms of being that prevent brothers from becoming dogs and teach us to practice human kinship—in a way, to create a world in which all are related, including animals—in the evanescent present, which is the best we can hope for in face of an inevitably violent future.

INTERLUDE

Standing at a Slight Angle to the Universe

One hot day in 2011 a man from OSACS (Odisha State AIDS Control Society) landed in Bhadrak to conduct a meeting with hijras in which he posed the question, "Who is a hijra?" The gathered hijras looked confused by the question, so he reformulated it to ask, "What kind of human beings are called hijras?" Lakshmi said, "In the whole of Bhadrak, I am the only hijra who is real (*asli*). I am the only one born from mother's stomach as a hijra." Lakshmi was referring to being born with genitalia that were not recognized as signifying either male or female, and this fact of being hijra by birth and not through castration accorded her a lot of respect. She considered every other hijra as false (*nakli*).

While I was interviewing Anto and Bhatto, I asked them how many kids they have, and after they answered, I asked them whether the kids were theirs. Anto answered an emphatic "yes." Shonali, who was sitting nearby, burst into laughter and said, "Look, with such pride she is saying she is the father of the children." That same evening, when we were returning from Anto and Bhatto's house, she suddenly said disgustedly, "Are they hijras? Producing three, four kids?—they're just *gandus*. Who would call them hijras?"[1] I asked her what a real hijra is, and she replied, "Those who don't marry and have children." Anto and Bhatto would not consider Jaina, Shamsheri, Azgari, Akhtari, or Mehraaj to be hijras because they did not wear saris but *lungis* (the sarong/loincloth worn by males). Jaina and the others would defend themselves by saying that since they didn't have to go begging on trains, they did not have to wear saris. Furthermore, Jaina explained that while she and her friends wore *lungis*, they always wore blouses, not *kurtas* (shirts worn by men), and carried *chunnis* (the flowing garment worn by women) instead of wrapping a towel around themselves like men. Jaina said definitively, "People who are in the know will know we are hijras by even the little hint of a slip of a towel; we don't need to wear saris like those prostitutes."

The guru of the Jajpur household of hijras used to often chastise her *celas* (followers or disciples) and *nati-celas* (followers of followers, or grand-followers, analogous with grandchildren) by screaming that they were not hijras but just *gandus* because they would take such a long time to get castrated. She would say, "It is a matter of great shame when people in the market see them and they have penises as large as elephants' trunks swinging between their legs." Meanwhile her celas would disdain Shonali and the hijras of Bhadrak because "they don't have a guru, they have not initiated themselves into a *gharana* (household), they are just *gandus* who beg on the trains." According to the Jajpur hijras, they had a right to beg on the train because they belonged to a proper hijra *gharana*.[2] Madhubai, who belonged to one of the oldest and most prestigious hijra *gharana* in eastern India, gave me her opinion. According to her, hijras of her house, and of other old and respected hijra houses in the country, hijras who beg on trains were not considered real hijras; the real hijras were those who collected money at weddings, childbirths, and other auspicious events such as the inauguration of a new shop, factory, or business venture.

The point to be taken here is that hijras' authenticity could not only be proven or disproven at multiple locations, but that those contextual criteria themselves were subject to contestation and calibration.[3] Lawrence Cohen, in his article "The Pleasures of Castration: The Postoperative Status of Hijras, Jankhas, and Academics," writes, "When I first started learning from and reading about *hijras*, I was struck by the centrality of the rhetoric of the false *hijra*, and of the power of this *hijra* insight in writing against the appropriation and misreading of the radically regendered body by those with perhaps less at stake." Cohen concludes this essay by arguing that instead of looking at noncastrated bodies as either "on the way" or as the bodies of "false" hijras, we might actually see it as "coherence to pleasures which grow out of [one's] community's performative traditions."[4] More than a decade later, Cohen offers a much more succinct explanation of the relation between *asli* and *nakli* hijras:

The anthropology of hijra life has tended to portray the relation between true hijras (who are intersexed or have had the operation, or have been accepted into the community by a hijra guru) and false hijras (who dress and dance as women but are not a third gender, or have not been accepted into the community) in terms of denunciation. But the border between authentic and inauthentic hijra embodiment, or belonging, is as much an improvisational exercise in creating a form of life under varied conditions of patronage and violence as it is a difference constitutive of sexual ethnicity.[5]

While Cohen disabuses us from seeking an authentic hijra, we are still left with the task of qualifying hijras' asceticism. I should hasten to add that hijras are not the only population whose asceticism is not easily discernible. Michael Carrithers, in his study of Buddhist ascetics of Sri Lanka, wrote, "One anthropologist was driven to describe the *sangha*'s salient characteristics as 'amorphousness,' by which I think he meant its perpetual division into small units—individual monks, single monasteries, or at most small groups of monks related by pupillary succession and only notionally attached to any larger group."[6] The same definition could aptly and accurately describe the way hijras organize themselves into households under gurus able to trace their belonging to one of the seven documented hijra *gharanas*. We can extend Das's argument about ascetics being able to force a relationship between themselves and God to claim that the ascetic lubricates the relationship among the various actors of the social—the king, the Brahman, and the householder—by the intensity of their ascetic practices.

In Chapters 1 and 2 I put forward the idea that hijras enter and participate in the social diagonally, following the tangential trajectory of a ray, touching but not crossing points. I find it an appropriate metaphor because if we take the tangent back to its mathematical roots in trigonometry, the ray is what forms a triangle. Hijra is located similarly and triangulates the duality of man and woman. If two points determine a line and three a plane, the demarcated difference is dependent on a third point, or planar surface; it is only through the third point that one can triangulate the distinction between the two points establishing a line, thus enabling man and woman to be determined as distinct locations as opposed to existing on a continuum.

The shorthand "third gender" affixed to hijras testifies to this triangulation and the tangent to the relationship they have to the opposite and the adjacent (sexes). In addition to this clarifying mathematical metaphor, I explored the relationship between the human and the animal as the interpretive valence of hijras' diagonal participation. I suggested that while she allows her lovers to become animal in the fucking fields to return as human to the domestic hearth, she allows her brothers to remain human instead of becoming the "animals" that householders do. Veena Das redraws the human-versus-animal distinction to domestic-versus-wild: the one is sacrificed and the other is hunted. Humans are seen related to *pashu* (domestic animals), and in making this shift, Das argues for a difference between nonviolence (*ahimsa*) and noncruelty (*anrhamsya*) to be taken seriously; for her, the difference gathers force "from the fact that a disposition is generated through the experience of togetherness."[7] The summary of Das's argument is that while the dharma of nonviolence disavows intimacy of any kind, the dharma of noncruelty arises from relationality. This difference is necessary because if one were to follow the rule of nonviolence strictly, one would not be able to live, since one would not be able to eat. The melancholia resulting from this inevitable loss and damnation is at least mitigated by noncruelty. One might be damned for living, but one's irrational affinities still have a force, an energy that makes one act caringly.

In Chapter 3, upcoming, I shall employ Das's argument concerning the noncruelty that is necessarily taught through our intimacy with animals to argue that hijras in some sites and moments becomes "the animal" to impart precisely this pedagogic lesson. Before proceeding, it may be helpful to revisit the debate that took place in the late 1950s between the anthropologists G. M. Carstairs and Morris E. Opler, in which the former maintained that hijras were male prostitutes while the latter argued they were ritual specialists.[8] That they are in actuality not only the one or the other, but arguably both at once, forces us to explicate the relationship between their eroticism and their asceticism that is both familiar and not. The figure who offers the clearest instance of the braiding of eroticism and asceticism is the Hindu god Shiva, as Wendy Doniger has argued; yet he can hardly serve as the exemplar for hijras, given that the economy of semen is reversed.[9] Shiva's asceticism, the retention of his semen, generates his eroticism and renders his semen fertile whenever and wherever he sheds it. For hijras, by contrast, the complementarity of eroticism and asceticism is not one of retention to make more fertile, but the opposite. They are ascetic not only in their abdication of shedding semen, ever, but also in the way they absorb and consume the semen of others. Their asceticism stems from their eroticism, whereas for Shiva, eroticism is the consequence of his ascetic practices. Doniger also notes that "these Indian ascetics are after power, not goodness—and they are after it for their own use; they *win* something, but they do not *grow into* anything; they possess something new, but who they are does not become something new. They exist in 'nontime' or 'collapsed time.'"[10]

We are thus obliged to look for a model of hijras' asceticism elsewhere; the work her asceticism achieves must be of some other kind if it is not making her seed more fertile. The "diagonal" definition being offered in the present study positions hijras as taking part in, or as an exemplar of, Lee Edelman's thesis of a nonheteronormative temporality (discussed in the introduction), and in so doing builds on the interpretive merit of the images invoked in the previous chapters. The diagonal entrance into the social—which allows for a relationship between the human-within-the-animal and the animal-within-the-human—in turn allows for respite from the social and preserves hijras' brothers and lovers for the world. This social formation allows a certain break in the heteronormative temporal unfolding of the life projects of householders. Chapter 4 of this volume will demonstrate how hijras' asceticism and eroticism make them live in what Doniger has called collapsed time.

What this "collapsed time" might offer and imply is hinted at by Sophie Day when she points out the similar temporal undulations of asceticism and eroticism in the lives of sex workers. She observes, "While many women [sex workers] sustained relationships with the world they had left over significant periods of time, they also abandoned the effort of stitching together the past and future with the present, the far away with the close at hand, and they joined an alternative counter-public."[11] Here Day adds that she is using the term "counter-public" "in reference to Warner's (2002) definition rather than Fraser's (1990), connoting a nonreproductive stance toward both biological and social reproduction."[12] Day further compares sex workers to religious ascetics, claiming that they share similar ideas of freedom that emerge from inhabiting such forms of collapsed time:

> Sex workers' views of freedom might be compared, however, to highly valued religious and secular practices of transcendence in the Western imagination such as those associated with solitary religious ascetics, performers, or competitive sports. Such values indicate that a sense of coer-

cion attaches inevitably, in our view, to the long-term relationships we inhabit. They show that our idioms of freedom delineate a non-relational and, at times, nonreproductive world as much as a social world of equals.[13]

The anthropology of hijras, I argue, offers us glimpses of what Edelman identifies as nonheteronormative temporality, and perhaps more importantly—as Chapter 4 will argue—it coheres with the sexuality proposed by Edelman, a sexuality articulated precisely via asceticism. This is not mere coincidence; these features of hijra existence belong together in complementarity. There is no need to contrast or reconcile asceticism and sex work because hijras are ascetics and sex workers at the same time, a conflation that seemed impossible for Carstairs and Opler to imagine. Finally, I offer a certain picture of the freedom that comes with this collapsed time, or nonheteronormative temporality. I argue that the life process, and thus time as experienced by hijras, can be seen as an unfolding of a mystical design, and although one cannot be aware of the final image or purpose of this design, it renders the present free from the weight of the past and the future or the "after" of sex as an open time of possibility, even if the actualization of that possibility is unimaginable.

3

SOMETHING ROTTEN IN THE STATE

Hijras in the district headquarters of Bhadrak, Jajpur, Balasore, Cuttack, and Khorda often fought amongst themselves regarding on which trains each group of hijras could beg. These fights—which would often turn physically violent—were resolved by hijras themselves by calling a committee of elder hijra gurus, who did not beg on the same trains, to arbitrate and pass judgment. The trains at the heart of these disputes plied the eastern coast of India between the cities of Guwahati and Hyderabad and went through Odisha railway stations at Balasore, Jalasore, Bhadrak, Jajpur, Cuttack, Khordha, and Bhubaneshwar. One confrontation was settled after it was decided the train called Falaknama Superfast Express would be divided in the following manner: Kanak and her *celas* (disciples) would beg on the train from Balasore to Bhadrak, while hijras from Bhadrak would beg on the train from Bhadrak to Cuttack, and hijras from Cuttack would beg on the train from Cuttack to Khordha. Since the passengers would not pay each group of hijras that would come aboard the trains in a single trip, the days of the week were divided, as well. Thus, one group would beg on that particular train on Monday, another group on Tuesday, another group on Wednesday, and so on until all the days that the train traveled were covered. Fighting would usually break out during the months when there were more days than groups, and each group would want to claim the extra day, or in other words, the extra train. Since Falaknama ran seven days a week, it was a particular bone of contention for hijras of Odisha.

Superfast or express trains that traveled between large cities were especially lucrative because they not only transported large numbers of passengers, but they carried passengers who were richer. Since the superfast and express trains span the distance between large metropolises and cater to a middle-class population in air-conditioned bogies (cars), hijras could coerce them to part with larger amounts of money—fifty rupees if the person was traveling alone, or ten rupees per person if there was a vacationing family. Thus a group of hijras might travel from their town of residence—for example, Bhadrak—and beg on the Falaknama going down to Cuttack on Tuesdays and Thursdays, then they might have to wait for a local train that ferries the local population between the state capital and the district headquarters. The riders of crowded local trains, usually the poorer rural population, would not part with their limited resources readily, and they were not as easily intimidated. Hijras might get at most five rupees per person. The fights would typically be over gaining control of the super-fast and express trains by the various groups of hijras. A usual day of earning money would consist of getting on a local or superfast express train early in the morning between 5:00 and 7:00 A.M., collecting money until the agreed-upon limit station—for hijras in Jajpur it would be Bhadrak, and for hijras in Bhadrak it would be Cuttack. After their stint on the train hijras of Jajpur, henceforth called the Jajpurias, would relax under some trees at the Bhadrak railway station, then take a local train back to Jajpur, begging as they went, where they would have lunch and a siesta, then repeat the procedure with two other trains in the evening from 6:00 to 11:00 P.M.

The recurrent fights would commonly break out in the Bhadrak railway station where the Jajpurias were relaxing. They were often accosted and attacked by hijras of Bhadrak, henceforth referred to as Bhadrakalis, if they had gone begging on trains that had not been assigned to them. Begging on somebody else's train would be called *gari maarna* (stealing the train), an easy and often-committed infraction. Even if the Jajpurias were assigned a train—for example, the Coromandel Express—it would have to run through Bhadrak first if it was going south, and the Bhadrakalis could easily get on that train by skipping lunch and taking a local train up to Balasore, collecting the money from the passengers from Balasore to Bhadrak, then getting off and hiding at home. Fights would also ensue if a power vacuum was perceived among hijra gurus. For instance, fights broke out when Kanak, the hijra guru based in Jaleswar, took on as her *celas* several hijras in Bhadrak who were without a guru till 2009, thereby increasing her authority over four districts in Odisha and challenging the once strong Jajpurias. In fact, Kanak even convinced several hijras from Jajpur to leave their guru and join her *gharana.*

When I reached the area to do fieldwork I asked Mangu, one of the Bhadrakalis, to take me on the trains with her, and she agreed. But when I reached the station she told me to come back another day and to wear a sari. She said I looked very unconvincing as a hijra in *salwaar kameez* (tunic and trouser outfit). When I came back a few days later in a sari, Mangu asked me whether I would be able to fight if the passengers refused to give money and created trouble. When I replied that I wouldn't, she looked a bit worried, and I sensed her reluctance; she said that she would take me on the local train later in the evening. While I was walking back I ran into the Jajpurias, who were having a snack while waiting for their train back. They said that they would take me begging on the trains: "We even take our lovers when they don't have money for their tickets. You are a hijra, we can take you easily, this is how we teach young hijras when they first come." After a week, I asked the guru of the Jajpur house to ask her *celas* to take me begging on the trains, and she told her *celas* in front of me, "Take her with you and ask with love and peace (*pyar aur santi*), don't start a fight." I got ready, and a group of us walked to the train station, but when the train arrived I found myself alone with a visibly miffed Lovely. I asked her what the matter was. She said, "Look, Guruma said she would take you on the train so she should have taken you. You are new, so you cannot fight or handle the passengers if they start to create trouble, so obviously, whoever goes with you will earn less because they will have to see how much they can take without creating any trouble. What if they fight, how will you protect yourself? Guruma should have taken you; she earns more than everybody else because we all give her a part of our earning every day. I don't mind taking you but I won't be able to earn that much alone, and they all left me, saying you are my friend so I should accept the responsibility. How will I earn? Why will the passengers give me money if I don't threaten them? Not even a mother feeds a child if the child doesn't cry."

Lovely fell silent. After a few minutes I said, "Listen, I don't want to create trouble and I won't be able to fight so why don't you go alone and I'll go home." I insisted on leaving, and since the train had arrived, Lovely didn't have much time to disagree. What had been glossed as begging in the literature I had read, and seemed such an obvious concept to translate, gradually began to unfold as an incredibly complex transaction. I finally went begging on the trains with Kanak, and this chapter's ethnography comes from those travels. Kanak pooh-poohed all my concerns about fighting and said she could handle everything; she has taught many hijras before. "Look at Paayal," she said, "she is now getting on trains without fear. When she first came, she would not say anything, would not ask anything, and would walk holding the hem of my sari, hiding behind me." I went begging ten times with Kanak and four times later with Biju and Anto before I had an accident that put an end to my begging on trains.

I should hasten to add that I am using the word *begging* here as a heuristic or as shorthand before taking it apart. The majority of the literature on hijras translates the transactions that take place on the trains between hijras and the passengers as begging, and there is some merit in using the word, since it introduces us to the broad category of economic exchange that is the mainstay of a hijra's income. I will complicate the use of the word, however, and further differentiate it from the way other economic transactions are seen and studied in order to argue that the way hijras talk about begging hints at a different corner of the moral economy. By moral economy I am referring to exchanges and transactions that include money changing hands but are necessarily mediated by notions of purity and pollution— and actors here include not only priests but also ancestral spirits, gods, and goddesses. Part of the moral economy is the economic relationship between the householder and the ascetic, or the king and the brahman, and across caste, that governs the status of the donor's body and soul. The next section will look at these circuits of exchange.

DANA, DAKSHINA, AND DALALI

One of the ways in which the issue of begging divided the community was emphatically repeated to me by hijras who were members of the traditional hijra *gharanas*. I met Dolly just once, but when she found out who my friends were, her face screwed up in disdain and disgust. She said, "We don't think they are hijras, those who beg on trains. They have no honor and are just *gandus*."[1] For hijras like Dolly, who belong to these old, respected, established hijra households with large numbers of *celas* and *nati-celas*, whose right to take money at weddings and childbirths was undisputed, even protected by the police, begging on trains was an activity that was shameful. Hijras who did beg on trains and were comfortable doing so would never use the term "begging" to describe what they did, which is what leads me to believe that begging is not the most fitting word for the transaction. Other hijras who would often express the shame they felt from begging were those who were skeptical about hijra communities' moral right to the money and yearned for a more secure source of income—as did Masterani, for example. Or they would—like Nandita, Damru, and Suman—feel ashamed of begging but not of earning money through sex work, where they said they had staked their bodies and "worked hard" to earn money.

Hijras who were considered—or accused of being—*nakli* or false because of begging on trains, and more recently at traffic signals, would disavow the shame through the use of the phrase *challa mangna*. They would say, "*X challa mangne gayi hai*" or "*gadi mangne gayi hai*" (she's gone to ask train).[2] The substitution of *challa* and *gaadi* with *bheek* (alms) would not require the grammatical structure of the sentence to be changed; it would read with substitution as "*X bheek mangne gayi hai*" (she's gone to ask for alms) or "*bheek mangne gayi hai*" (she's gone begging). While there is no syntactical dissonance created with the substitution, a semantic difference is highlighted with the use of *bheek*. First of all, nobody ever said, *bheek mangne gayi hai* (she's gone begging) upon casual inquiry about a person's whereabouts. *Bheek* was used by hijras such as Dolly who sought to assert their authenticity and denounce the falseness of other hijras. Nandita, Damru, and Suman used it to make their discomfort felt in asking for money that they did not feel they had earned through hard work. Suman would say, "I feel very ashamed to ask for *bheek*; why should I ask them, when God has given me a body, I can work hard and eat. They [the passengers] might also wonder and ask—why should we give her money when she has her hands and feet." Finally, *bheek* was used by Masterani to associate the shame of begging with its instability. She was looking for a job with an NGO, and when I told her that salaries don't come frequently or on time at NGOs, she acceded to my point but didn't revise her position on begging—the insecure income of a respectable job seemed more appealing to her than the secure income of a shameful activity.

Let me give an instance of the semantic difference between the use of the word *challa* and *bheek* as it became clear through the explicatory use of the word *haq*. Some activists from Bangalore and New York visited an NGO office in the district headquarter town of Bhadrak to talk to some hijras. Lovely, Jaina, Anto, Bhatto, a few others, and I were asked to come talk to them. I will not analyze the conversation here, but on hearing the fact that one of them was a lawyer, Lovely asked, "Do hijras have the *haq* to ask for *challa* on the trains or not?" (*hijra log ko train mein challa mangne ka haq hai ki nahin hai?*). The lawyer who had come from Bangalore answered that according to India's laws, hijras do not have the right to beg for money. Lovely looked highly unconvinced but didn't say anything in reply and tuned out of the rest of the conversation. The reason Lovely looked unconvinced at the lawyer's answer is that, regardless of the colonial and modern history of policing and criminalizing hijras in public spaces, the practice of collecting *challa* (begging on trains), *badai* (begging at weddings and childbirth), and performing at religious festivals in public spaces has persisted. The failure to police and discourage hijras from practicing their occupations resonates with the failure of contemporary efforts to make hijras more respectable in terms of their economic activity. It could be argued that the failure to police hijras can primarily be attributed to the fractured nature of colonial policing and governmentality.[3] Without either bolstering or discounting this argument, I want to suggest that there is another reason hijras themselves have persisted in collecting money through performances, blessings, and curses in the public space. This insistence on the right to collect money—as expressed by Lovely—can be understood only through the notion of *haq*, which not only renders what they do on trains different from begging but also implies different stakes in giving up such a right. This argument becomes clearer when we look at what hijras are willing to do to collect the money they believe rightly belongs to them.[4]

One day Rekha was removing a large pin from her sari. When I asked why she used such a large one, she said, "If there is ever a fight on the train, to protect ourselves we can take a pin out and poke them." She also told me that that morning a young man traveling on the train told her that he did not have any change; she promised to give him change after she had finished collecting money from the rest of the bogie. He handed over a five-hundred rupee note, and she tucked it in her blouse and ran off without returning the change she had promised. Rekha ended her account by asking, "Why should I give back the money that belongs to hijras?" (*hijralog ka paisa wapas kyon denge?*). Hijras' sense that the money collected on trains properly belongs to them, just as the citizen's tax payment properly belongs to the state, forces one to read *challa* not so much as part of the moral circuit of begging, which I shall discuss later, but in terms of ethical payment of taxes to which they have a right, or *haq*.

The third incident that suggested to me that collecting *challa* is similar to collecting taxes took place on a train traveling between Bhadrak and Jaleswar. Kanak and I had gone begging one day; after making our way through the train, we reached the last of the second-class bogies. Hijras are not allowed by the police to beg in first class. Moreover, the first-class compartments are usually cordoned off so that one cannot hop from a second-class bogie to first-class cars. I had stayed behind at the entrance of the last second-class car to take notes, waiting for Kanak to return to me, given that it was the last "open" bogie. I saw a man step out of the loo and, on seeing Kanak, he exclaimed, "Arre baba!" (Oh God!) and went back to hide in the loo. Kanak came back and asked the man's friend to give her some money; when he refused, she abused him and physically harassed him by throwing her body's full weight on his lap. The friend emerged from the loo and said, "I don't like them at all, they take money from you by force, and if you don't give it to them, they abuse you." What struck me as similar about collecting *challa* and collecting taxes in this case was the way in which the man evaded Kanak. He, like the other passengers, did not question *why* hijras should be given money but simply tried to get out of or escape paying them. I shall build on this subtle difference to qualify the logic of exchange that took place between hijras and the passengers. Also, what seemed odd was the manner in which the man felt threatened by the abuses and light physical harassment—when he could have retaliated blow by blow and overpowered the hijra with the help of his fellow passengers.

I want to begin analyzing the transactions on the train by comparing them with *dana*. According to Maria Heim, *dana* can be translated as gift, generosity, gift-giving, alms, and hospitality, and it "describes a key religious practice of making merit as well as a central social value of hospitality widely affirmed in South Asian religion."[5] Jonathan Parry has argued in his essay "On the Moral Perils of Exchange" that the passing of sins is central to a certain set of economic exchanges in Hinduism and affects various other forms of exchanges that constitute the economy of the local moral and economic world of Benares. *Dana* as understood by Parry is the gift given to the funerary priests who perform rituals to transform "the malevolent ghosts of the unincorporated dead (*preta*)" and rituals toward "the incorporated ancestors (*pitras*)."[6] Given that the ideal moral transaction entailing the priest giving away what he received as *dana* "with increment" (because as a renouncer he cannot concern himself with accumulation of wealth) is impossible, the exchanges between the priest and the donor offer us a glimpse of how the moral person is split to facilitate an economy. There are two moral-temporal orders at work here: those of *artha* and *dharma*.

> The term *artha* refers not only to the realm of politico-economic power which is the third of the four conventionally enumerated goals of human existence, but more generally also has the sense of "means." Thus *artha*, as material and coercive power, is the "means" by which man may attain the sensual delights of *kama* and sustain the moral order of *dharma*. What Hindu thought rejects is that these means should become the ultimate end. *Artha* must be pursued in conformity with the hierarchically superior dictates of *dharma*. . . . The strict disjunction between the two realms—and the thoroughgoing ideological subordination of the politico-economic domain—cuts it loose from its moral moorings and deprives it of real meaning. . . . Denied "the slightest value or intellectual interest," almost anything goes; and to a significant extent it is this devaluation which condemned the Indian polity to perpetual instability. By only a slight extension of the same argument, we can see that commerce suffers a similar semantic impoverishment, and the condemnation of its abuses is consequently robbed of real force. Emptied of moral content it cannot be a major source of moral peril.[7]

So, for example, while the transactions that the priest conducts are beset with moral peril (they have to digest the sins of the donor and the death pollution of the dead), the transactions of the trader are not, because "the acquisition of commercial wealth is a legitimate and laudable objective, but it is one that is ultimately justified by the generosity with which it is then disbursed." The acquisition of wealth through rapacious and unscrupulous means is allowed for the trader because it is his *jati-dharma*, his code of conduct, but he too must eventually dispose of the wealth by giving it to the priest to cleanse himself of sins. Parry reminds us that the king, too, like the trader, is split: "The traditional Indian is recognized as having much in common with the bandit; and it is by violence, conquest and plunder that he is supposed to fund the sacrifice, or the gifts which replace it."[8]

The orders of *dharma* and *artha* are relevant because they will determine the legitimacy of hijras' right to collect money from passengers in trains—

mostly coercively, but not always. For the present, I cite Parry's work to differentiate *dana* from hijras' collection of *challa*, which does not tie in with the circuit of moral perils. The *dana* that the Mahabrahman priests in Benares were collecting came with a certain moral charge of expunging the sins of the donor; no such meaning was ever referred to by hijras in relation to *challa*. Parry's ethnography makes the point that the priest cannot pass on the *dana* with an added increment because not only does he have to provide for his family, he also has no other source of income; thus the dual temporal orders of morality—of *artha* and *dharma*—result in the priest's failure to follow a rule.[9] Jenny Huberman, whose research was also based in Benares, has written on the young boys and girls who work as tour guides for foreign visitors, comparing the moral perils of *dana* as Parry has studied it with the *dalali* that the young people did. She translates *dalali* as "both the business of commission or brokerage work and the commission itself."[10] Huberman's ethnography argues that *dalali* or commercial work was morally perilous as well, similar in some ways to the *dana* that Parry has studied. Huberman's drawing of these similarities troubles the divide between *artha* and *dharma*—a divide that both anthropologists have noted to be unclear in the first place, given that *artha* and *dharma* have a bearing upon each other. Though this may seem a moot point, it has implications that qualify what kind of earning is justified, which in turn is relevant to analyzing the legitimacy of collecting *challa*.

Huberman notes the following similarities between *dana* and *dalali*. The first is that the money earned from both forms of exchange is barren: "Like the proceeds of *dan*, the commissions (*dalali*) these boys earned were also described as forms of 'bad' (*galat*) or 'barren' money—people in the neighborhood of Dasashwamedh frequently maintained that they could not save this money or put it to productive use."[11] The barrenness of the money stemmed from the fact that it was polluted by the sinful manner in which it was earned. Given that the way the young boys earned the money "seemed a far cry from the work world of the *ghats*, where the Mallah livelihoods were secured with calloused hands and physical labour," the money earned through *dalali* was "talked about as a kind of unearned income, qualitatively different from the money of hard work (*mehnat ka paisa*)."[12]

Huberman's point in outlining these similarities is that money earned from *dalali* or commercial work had the potential to become polluted and barren just like *dana*—but the analogy breaks down. *Dana* carries with it the sins of the giver to be purified by the Brahmans, whereas none of the tourists who conducted economic exchanges in Huberman's ethnography were suffering from death pollution. While Huberman might be correct in pointing out the similarity in the barrenness of the money collected through *dana* and *dalali*, Parry himself locates the difference between these transactions elsewhere. Using the notion of the gift as studied by Marcel Mauss, he writes, "Where we have the 'spirit' reciprocity is denied; where there is reciprocity there is not much evidence of 'spirit.'"[13] In other words, the effect of pollution on the money that is accrued through *dana* and *dalali* might be the same, but the sites of the pollution are different: In the case of *dana*, it is the death pollution that the priest has to ingest, while for *dalali* it is the pollution of the immoral transactions that the youth undertake. My purpose in offering such an extensive elaboration is to differentiate *challa* from both *dana* and *dalali*. None of the aforementioned kinds of arguments concerning pollution were even remotely raised in connection with *challa*, either by hijras or by the men of Bhadrak who traveled on those trains weekly to Calcutta to collect goods to be sold in the village market. The money collected was never seen as tainted, polluted, or barren, even though hijras sometimes cheated and often coerced the passengers. The reason for this was that the money, according to all the hijras I ever spoke to, rightly belonged to them, and the passengers, in refusing or hesitating to give them the money, were the ones cheating.

Hijras worked very hard to earn their money, getting up at the crack of dawn to prepare themselves to jump on the trains. Getting ready entailed bathing, putting on makeup, wearing clean, gaudy saris, and hiding large pins, in case a stubborn passenger got violent. It was also labor performed in the wake of negotiating a form of being, which is bound to the train itself. Since the trains stopped in Jajpur and Bhadrak early in the morning, hijras would first commute from their home to the town where their jurisdiction had been allotted, then take another train back. They would briefly have lunch and rest, get on another train in the late afternoon, then travel back home from the allocated town. They would return to have dinner and crash, only to repeat the entire journey the next day. Since collecting *challa* meant they would pass through all the compartments, they were always on their feet and rarely paused for rest. Neither were they whimsical regarding the frequency with which they went to collect *challa*; they dutifully got up and went to collect every day, and when they missed the train because it was hard to get out of bed on early winter mornings, they would sulk and say, "I missed the train." In fact, the tight schedule hijras followed made conducting fieldwork very difficult initially because they had little free time to lounge about and chat with me. It was only when I started traveling with them on the trains that I realized how packed and exhausting their working days were. When not riding the trains, they were cooking, scrubbing dirty dishes, washing clothes, or mending their houses. The hard work they did was implicit not only in their schedules but also in the manner that senior hijras blessed the junior hijras: whenever a *cela* wanted to go settle somewhere else, if the hijra guru allowed it, she would give her blessing by saying *khato aur khao*—"work hard and eat."

This blessing would be used in different circumstances, as well; for example, if a *cela* wanted to leave her hijra guru's house, she would have to pay a fine and then would be blessed, *khato aur khao*, and allowed to leave. Hijras would often proclaim their legitimacy by saying, "We don't eat at the mercy of somebody else, we work hard and eat" (*humlog kisi ka nahin khaate hai, khat ke khate hai*). Thus, the money collected was seen as earned through hard work, neither as tainted with the sins of the passengers nor as accreting pollution or barrenness by being earned in this manner. *Challa* is also only partially similar to the set of essential and caste-based forms of ritual labor such as midwifery or funerary broadly known as *jajmani*. Even though hijras would often refer to shopkeepers and other tradesman as *jajman*, a crucial difference emerged because hijras cut across caste lines.[14] If harm was caused in the process of earning, it was because their *haq* was being breached or they were being denied what they saw as rightfully belonging to them. While the money earned was not seen as transferring pollution, the hijra in some ways was similar to the brahman in that she could influence the relationship between god and the householder—by cursing the men with impotence or childlessness or even death to the householder's children in default of an exchange of money. This partial similarity between hijras and the brahman rotates around the figure of the *sanyasi*, the ascetic renunciate who is sometimes structurally opposed to the brahman and sometimes parallel to him, as we shall see when we return to this shortly.[15]

The hard work that goes into collecting *challa* is not what prevents it from being recognized as a form of begging. James Staples has remarked on the long hours of labor in begging undertaken by lepers in less than salubrious conditions that included inclement weather and hostile police. I want to juxtapose the begging undertaken by lepers as studied by James Staples with the collecting of *challa* as undertaken by hijras, not only to draw on similarities—which would qualify hijras as ascetic figures because they feel they are deserving of a share of the other person's earnings—but also on differences that distinguish them from lepers and other recipients of *dakshina*. *Dakshina* is a supplement to *dana*, not always synonymous, and is given to various figures associated with the temple economy, such as lepers.[16] *Dakshina* denotes "the end of the cycle of activities" associated with sacrificial voyage and terminates the relationship between the priest and the householder/king. Only after the *dakshina* is given is the person who authorized the sacrifice allowed to "take the fruits of the action."[17]

The deformed body of the leper is crucial in legitimizing begging, and the deformity can be exaggerated in the theatrically performed act of begging to elicit more pity and gain higher earnings. James Staples writes, "The recognizable effects of leprosy socially legitimated the use of their bodies in practice, like begging, that elicited moral disapprobation outside the context of religious mendicancy. . . . People knew that they could enhance their earnings as beggars by exposing the physical signs of leprosy, but this was seen as compensation for the affliction they had suffered."[18] The body of hijras, even when not seen as deformed, played as crucial a role in extracting money from passengers on the train. Paayal told me that when she goes on the train, the young boys would often tease and ask, "Sister, how come you don't have breasts?" (*Didi, aapke chaati kyon nahin hai?*) Paayal would clap her hands and reply, "If hijras had breasts, what would be the use of having girls in this world?" The body of hijras would often result in puzzlement rather than pity. I was often asked by random strangers who had been informed by shopkeepers that I lived with hijras, "Is the top part of their body female and the lower part male, or is the lower part of the body female and the top part male? Do they have a hole down there but cannot produce children?" Hijra bodies are also put on display when collecting *challa* by being wrapped in gaudy saris and decked in jewelry. In addition to the clothes and jewelry, hijras' bodies announce themselves by the distinctive clapping called *thigri* and the threatening assertiveness of the voice, loudly demanding money—no obsequious beseeching for alms here.[19] But this threatening stance is calibrated according to other influencing factors, such as the strength that comes from begging in numbers. Let me explain this further.

One evening Bhatto, Anto, Varsha, and I were drinking. Bhatto started recounting how, when they would get bored on the trains while begging or when they would not get as much money as they wanted, they would start pretending that they had severe physical deformities—not only to laugh at the passengers recoiling in disgust but also to increase their collection. Amidst loud peals of laughter from everybody, Bhatto showed how people would screw their faces in repulsion and terror when Meena Kisu and Bhatto would walk with an exaggerated limp or crawl on their hands. Given that they would also be highly inebriated, Bhatto laughed and showed how Meena and Varsha would jut out their faces, smelling of country hooch, into the passengers' faces and make loud indecipherable noises to make them part with their money quickly. While hijras could and would grab the balls of young men to make them part with money, they were quite at a loss as to how to deal with middle-aged men if they were not begging in a large group. One of the tactics passengers routinely used to discourage hijras from pressing for money was to take an inordinately long time to desist from whatever they were doing, look for their wallet, take it out, then begin to gather the paltry amount of money they were willing to give—looking for their loose change, counting it, then finally handing it over. With many bogies to go through, hijras would get very irritated at these tactics and ask the stalling men to hurry up, but they knew they could only intimidate these men if they were begging in a large group. The older the man was, the less threatened he felt by hijras, probably because he was already a father or grandfather and threats of impotence were ineffective for him. These men were also capable of creating a ruckus; if a hijra became too aggressive or violent in her demands, they would often grab hold of her, beat her up, and complain to the train conductor with whom hijras had tacit agreements on how to beg.

While displaying the body and performing the deformity is partially similar between lepers and hijras, the possibility of violence differentiates it. Staples notes, "When a benefactor does not fulfill the expected criteria, the beggar also reserves the right to go elsewhere. For example, few of Bethany's beggars now visited the Jain businessman who gave away food packets and cash incentives because, as one informant put it, 'he expects us to eat the food there and wait around a while.' In the time that it takes to consume what he has to offer, an individual could have secured greater gains through conventional begging."[20] While lepers would decide not to create a ruckus, hijras who begged on trains would be prepared for fights, especially if they were traveling in a large group. Anto, Bhatto, Varsha, and Meena Kisu were hijras of Bhadrak who would go begging together but would fan out and work individually to cover all the bogies. Consequently, they would have to be careful not to start a fight, given that they would not stand a chance if the passengers decided to gang up on them. This also explains why they would pretend to have physical deformities or mental health problems and replace the threat of physical coercion and violence with the threat of pollution and disgust—using a strategy similar that of the lepers—so as to not anger passengers. Hijras of Jajpur who belonged to a traditional *gharana* would go collecting *challa* in a large group of twenty, and when they fanned out throughout the train they made sure nobody begged alone in a bogie. They did not need to rely on disgusting the passengers into giving money, and they often went a step further by tricking passengers into giving more than they wanted.

In addition to the large pins hijras kept hidden in their saris, hijras would sometimes get carried away and stun passengers with hard slaps when they were being difficult. As Chandni would frequently get into fights that would threaten to erupt into a lot of physical violence, she was often urged to control her anger and keep calm; in such instances, the other hijras would beg forgiveness and fall on the feet of the passengers. The passengers were not always helpless when threatened by hijras. Once I was called by Lovely to come to the Railway Police Station in Bhadrak, where I found her in tears and nursing a sprained elbow. The story I gathered went as follows: Hijras from Bhubaneshwar had "stolen" the train from hijras of Jajpur and tried to force some young man to give them more money. When he refused they caught hold of him and roughed him up; he started bleeding from a wound to his head. When hijras from Jajpur, ignorant of what had occurred, got on the train to rightfully collect their *challa*, the passengers caught them and beat them up, even though they argued that they were innocent of beating the young man. The passengers, refusing to believe them, handed them to the railway policeman in Bhadrak, who looked even more harried when I appeared on the scene.

The possibility of violence on the part of both hijras and passengers marks the difference between collecting *challa* and begging and brings us closer to understanding the way in which hijras exhibited a certain logic of extraction. The possibility of violence existed because of the notion of *haq*—

translated as *rights*—that hijras felt they had to the money. While their *haq* was not disputed by the passengers, the *amount* of money that hijras claimed a right to was often questioned. Once, late in the evening, I had just alighted from the train in which I was begging when a young lad of seventeen came up to me. I had often seen him roaming around the bazaar, so I smiled. He said, "Please tell your friend to not trouble me, she is very naughty. If I give her five rupees, she will ask for ten and when you don't give it to her, she will do a lot of *badmaashi*; she will sit on you, pinch you, she once even slapped my friend." I was very touched by this polite request. By that time my friend, Kanak, had joined me from the other side of the train (she had taken the second-class, air-conditioned bogies and I the general class). I told her, "Kanak, don't take money from this boy anymore." Kanak looked disinterested, said, "Why shouldn't I take money from him?" and walked away. I shrugged my shoulders helplessly at the lad and left.

BHIKSHA AND HAQ

Collecting *challa*, I have noted, is only partially similar to other forms of monetary exchange. Let us consolidate this by further distinguishing *challa* from *bhiksha*, the daily begging of Buddhist monks. Michael Carrithers, in his study on Buddhist monks, mentions that the manner in which the *bhikkhu* begs is central to the aspiration and attainment of Buddhist asceticism—to the extent that the *bhikkhu* cannot ask, let alone coerce, anybody to give him his alms or daily meal—and "the basic framework of the day is founded on the necessity of begging and eating the main meal before noon."[21] Although hijras do not collect *challa* without coercion, they do organize their everyday life around that activity, as described earlier. Their insistence on their right (*haq*) to collect money qualifies their asceticism, to be sure, but the manner in which they conduct their begging requires more attention.[22]

To understand the labor performed by the ascetic we must look more closely at the notion of *bhiksha*. Carrithers in his work has insisted that the difference between Buddhist and Jain ascetics lies in the exchange that takes place between the ascetic and the laity: "There is no prescription that the *muni* owes anything to the laity, not even the 'gift of the Teaching,' which the Buddhist *bhikkhu* owes the Buddhist laity. *Munis* do, of course, participate in the relationships de facto, but it is important to stress that such relationships are not recognized in the conception of the *muni* in the formal language of Jains concerning *munis*. Relationships, in other words, are irrelevant to the *muni*'s defining characteristic, self-mortification."[23] He clarifies this relationship as one of dependence but not of reciprocity: "To receive such alms (but not give anything in return) is indeed the *munis*' only formal and prescribed interaction with the laity."[24] Hijras are similar to the Buddhist *bhikkhu* to the extent that their day and their asceticism are both qualified through begging, but different from them because they offer no services otherwise: no officiating ceremonies, teachings, or the like. In this respect they are similar to the Jain monks because while they lay a claim to the money, they are not expected to give anything in return. But given that the Jain monks, *munis*, cannot ask for money, let alone coerce the laity into giving them anything, hijras continue to differ from them. The coercion that hijras practice stems from their displaying their bodies in a way that is sometimes parallel and sometimes identical to the begging that lepers undertake. Hijras, as I have mentioned, when not strong in numbers would pretend to be deformed; but lepers, by contrast with hijras, are not aggressive in their deformity, pretended or real. More importantly, as Staples's ethnography has shown, lepers are expected to expiate the sins of the almsgiver. Thus the relationship between them is one of reciprocity, which is not the case with hijras.

The partial similarity that hijras' logic of extraction has to *dana*, *dakshina*, *dalali*, and *bhiksha* can be understood in the same vein as their participation in the social and the domestic, discussed earlier. The image of the arc, its diagonal entrance, and tangential trajectory, with which I have studied hijras' position in the social sphere, can also be applied to understand their logic of extraction and their participation in the moral economy of South Asia. While their begging touches all the aforementioned prescriptive types of exchange tangentially, it is not fully congruent with any of them.

Veena Das defines the Hindu *sanyasi* (ascetic) in a way that differentiates it from Buddhist and Jain asceticism: "Thus, while the king has political power, the *sanyasi* can acquire esoteric power, which can be transformed into political power."[25] But this does not locate the logic of extraction that hijras practice. Hijras do use their asceticism to make a political point in a quite literal sense—as the next sections of this chapter shall document—but they do not square easily with the *sanyasi* that Das depicts. As Das notes, "The renunciatory ideal followed by the *sanyasi* in the Dharmaranya Purana and in other Puranic texts is one which stresses a complete independence of the *sanyasi* from the world of the householder." While transforming their acquired power into political power and walking away from kingship, as the myth Das studies illustrates, hijras do not abandon the world at all. On the contrary, in fact, hijras call upon the world to give up money upon which they claim their right (*haq*).

The notion of *haq* justifies the threat of violence on the part of hijras. The passengers also implicitly assume it inasmuch as no one denies hijras their right to the money, even when they try not to part with it. The use of the word *haq* not only gives hijras a right to the money of the passengers, but also lays on them a responsibility that they cannot shirk—in this *challa* is similar to *jajmani* but is without the determining element of caste, which is crucial for distributing the variety of work that is provided to the *jajman* (patron). Hijras' use of the word *haq* to defend their asking for *challa* also helps to explain why various attempts made by well-meaning people to employ hijras in different professions have failed. Spivak, who has written on the difficulty of translating *haq*, comes closest when she writes, "*Haq* is the 'para-individual structural responsibility' into which we are born—that is, our true being. Indeed, the word 'responsibility' is an approximation here. For this structural positioning can also be approximately translated as birthright. Whether it is right or responsibility, it is the truth of my being, in a not quite English sense, my *haq*."[26] The prefix *para-* in Spivak's definition explains why hijras would lament their fate, which had doomed them to collect money at weddings, childbirths, religious festivals, and on trains in spite of the violence they would or could face. They lament because it is inescapable; not to collect *challa* would be to give up one's *haq* and consequently the truth of one's being. It also explains why passengers did not question the appropriateness of giving over money; this was not because of the threat of physical injury, for as we have seen, passengers too can gang up on hijras.

Spivak, like hijras, invokes *haq* to imagine a different mode of exchange, one other than begging, and one not determined by violence, when she writes, "Imagine yourself and them—as both receivers and givers—not in a Master-Slave dialectic, but in a dialogic of accountability."[27] Spivak's invocation of *haq* arises out of the contemporary moment of unequal exchanges in which accountability is forgone. Based on the ethnographic scenes on the trains, we learn from hijras what Spivak has asked us to learn: not only what exchange is in the current moment, but what it should be—a dialogic of accountability. Spivak further reflects, "Without an education into an epistemic transformation whose most efficient description I happen to find in *haq*, capital—industrial and finance—cannot be persistently checked and turned around to the interest of the social as practically laid out in the Marxian passage, which has not grown old. I am further arguing that this social practice of responsibility based on an imperative imagined as intended from alterity cannot today be related to any named grounding—as in Kant or Islam."[28] Hijras' *haq* educated the passengers on the trains, the citizens of the state, and the state governing its people as to how capital can be "persistently checked and turned around to the interest of the social." The form of checking and transforming capital that hijras conduct is minuscule within the larger scale of global capitalism, but it is the most familiar exchange, given that it takes place every day for a large population that travels on trains.

Hijras who belonged to a *gharana* and begged in large groups were able to collect a tidy sum. Reddy remarks in a footnote, "It is difficult to talk of class and to place hijras in a particular class based on income, the 'traditional' parameter for this differentiation. . . . In terms of actual income, hijras probably qualify as upper-middle-income or at least middle-income people, which ordinarily connotes a very different lifestyle—equivalent to that of a semi affluent middle-class—than the one they live. Judging by their lifestyle, they would probably be classed as low-income/lower-class."[29] This discrepancy between the class implied by the monthly income of hijras and the class implied by the privileges they inhabit not only reveals the terrain of gender and caste at play when trying to transform financial capital into social and cultural capital, but also raises the question of where money can go—or, in other words, the futurity implied by capital.

The money hijras earned would inevitably go to their family, even while they complained about the greediness of their family members. Though hijras claimed that family members only used them for their money and did not actually love them, the money would find its way to meet the expenditures of the family. Hijras neither thought of saving or of investing, at least not at the cost of refusing money to their family members. They would give money for medical treatments of their aging parents, tuition and college fees for their brothers and sisters, and clothes and presents for various occasions. They would shoulder a large part of the expenditure for the weddings of their nieces, nephews, younger brothers, and sisters. While this is where the money collected through begging by lepers would go as well, the difference lay in the position of hijras in the family. Staples notes that the large amount of money earned through begging enabled lepers "to reclaim some of the status their leprosy had cost them." One of his informants claimed, "The people in his village cared less about his deformities and saw him as a 'big man' to whom 'the Gods have shown favour,' all as a direct result of his economic prowess."[30] This transformation never took place for hijras; they never accreted respect because of their economic advantage. This failure to transform financial into social or cultural capital for hijras was not solely because of the source of their income. Staples showed that even when the villagers and neighbors of the leper knew that they earned their money through begging, they did not ever address it or raise it as an issue; in fact, begging was never mentioned, and instead ambiguous terms and phrases were used to address questions regarding the leper's livelihood, something that Staples refers to as a *language of concealment*.

Hijras in Bhadrak and Bhawanipatna, on the other hand, were always keenly aware of the sharp risk that they might bring shame onto their families through their very existence, even while their money was being used to ward off other potentially shame-inducing events. I want to press the irony of these circumstances. Bodies considered impotent, incapable, and damaged for the social like the hijra's—and the leper's to some extent— were in fact providing the labor and capital for the sustenance and transformation of bodies that are capable, potent, and fit for reproductive heteronormativity. I am not exactly arguing that the roles of impotency and potency are reversed here, but that people do not appear to be what they are; that, in short, we live in the era of *kalyug*, in which nothing is what it seems or should be.

THE HIJRA TAX COLLECTOR

Before we move on to a discussion of *kalyug*, I want to argue that the logic of extraction hijras operate on, understood through the notion of *haq*—with partial similarity to a host of other moral-economic exchanges—signals a logic of noncruelty. As we have just seen, Spivak invokes *haq* as accountability in a context of unequal exchanges in which accountability is forgone. This forgoing of accountability is what defines the relationship between the state and the public, which is why the electorate votes hijras into office and why they are recruited by the state to mark the corruption of exchange/accountability between the state and its citizens. The remainder of this chapter will discuss this phenomenon.[31] The logic of extraction that hijras exert is acknowledged by the state in several ways. The first is through the recruitment of hijras to collect taxes. The BBC carried an article in 2006 entitled "India Eunuchs Turn Tax Collectors." Here I quote the report in full so that we have a clear narrative against which to set up its various further iterations across newspapers and online news channels:

Tax authorities in one Indian state are attempting to persuade debtors to paying their bills—by serenading them with a delegation of singing eunuchs.

Eunuchs are feared and reviled in many parts of India, where some believe they have supernatural powers.

Often unable to gain regular employment, the eunuchs have become successful at persuading people to part with their cash.

The eunuchs will get a commission of 4% of any taxes collected.

In Bihar's capital, Patna, officials felt deploying the eunuchs was the only way to prompt people to pay up.

"We are collecting taxes for the municipal corporation, collecting money from those who have not paid their taxes for years," said Saira, one of the eunuchs on the streets of Patna.

"Tax payment is necessary. When the corporation won't have any money how will they look after the people?"

Accompanied by police officers, the eunuchs approached shopkeepers and large defaulters on their first foray into tax collection.

"Pay the tax, pay the Patna Municipal Corporation tax," the eunuchs sang as they approached Ram Sagar Singh, who owed 100,000 rupees (£1,180), the AFP news agency reported.

Mortified by the commotion, Mr. Singh reportedly agreed to pay up within a week.

The eunuchs collected about 400,000 rupees on their first day of work, authorities said, sharing 16,000 rupees (£188) amongst themselves.

Bharat Sharm, a revenue officer, told the Associated Press agency he was pleased with the eunuchs' work.

"We are confident that their reputation and persuasive skills will come in handy," he said.[32]

The news report was repeated across the channel by *USA Today* under the title "India Unleashes Eunuchs on Tax Cheats." The verb *unleashes* brings forth an image of a weapon or a pet monster, and this allusion is further cemented when we read about how the state is at its wit's end in trying to collect taxes. The *USA Today* article goes on to report, "20 eunuchs in bright saris began going from shop to shop, asking the owners to pay overdue municipal taxes in Patna, the capital of Bihar, one of India's most impoverished and lawless states" where the "city's tax arrears ran into the millions" and where "only 2000 of . . . nearly half million residents regularly pay property taxes and water charges." The municipal administrator, Atul Prasad, states, "Tax collection has slipped to 200 million rupees ($4.34 million) a year from the anticipated 700 million rupees ($15.2 million)." The report also warns readers "the eunuchs will be asked to help collect outstanding taxes from private homes soon."[33]

Almost a decade before the Bihar state municipality thought of commissioning hijras to collect taxes, a foreign bank operating in India had commissioned them as debt collectors. The *Sydney Morning Herald* of Australia reported on June 14, 1997, under the title "Gender-Benders Give Debtors Dressing Down to Make Them Pay Up; India's Repo 'Men.'" The news report reads, "When a foreign bank operating in India found recently that traditional methods were not succeeding in recovering bad debts, they turned to a secret new weapon: cross-dressers hurling abuse." Hijras are reported as "threatening to snatch or curse children unless protection money was paid. . . . Their vile insults and innuendos persuade many well-heeled families to cough up, such is the psychological power of the 'third sex.'" This article reveals what kind of weapon hijras are imagined by the state to be; like a cobra that has been defanged but is not known to be so, they are scary and *appear* lethal.[34]

Though the article cautions against confusing the metaphor with reality, I must mention another newspaper report—this time from across the border in Pakistan—to underline that while hijras are seen as a weapon, the state is using them precisely because it is trying *not* to harm its citizens. The *Guardian* carried a newspaper report entitled "Pakistan's Tax Dodgers Pay When the Hijra Calls," in which Qazi Aftab, the head of tax collection for the Clifton cantonment board in Karachi, identifies hijras' "clapping, shouting and generally making a scene" as "the nuclear option." The journalist Jon Boone reports, "The authorities are extremely pleased with their efforts to combat the tax dodgers. Aftab says recovery rates are up 15% from when conventional tax collectors often clashed violently with the householders. That never happens with the hijras, he said."[35] Apart from tax collection, hijras are also used by the state to fight crime and "clean up" Bombay,[36] to improve the birth and death registration rates,[37] and to improve border security. These projects of the state, I emphasize, are more spectacles for the media than even remotely serious suggestions to improve state governance. Furthermore, they borrow and feed into an idea of the past when hijras/eunuchs were respected and given powerful positions.[38]

In an essay, Veena Das argues that the power wielded by men as the holders of the state is made vulnerable in the light of the sexuality of the woman, because these men are also bearers of desire.[39] Here I want to borrow from Das the idea that the ethical imperative of this vulnerability is one of noncruelty rather than nonviolence. I want to position these scenes in which hijras are recruited as tax collectors, birth registration officials, and border security guards as scenes of the vulnerable state. This is confirmed by the way in which hijras are defined as weapons—as poisonless cobras or nuclear weapons pointed at citizens—that do not inflict the damage that actual nuclear weapons might. The fact that the state has other options to pursue all these problems yet chooses hijras not only relies on the logic of extraction that they offer, but also on a method that does not result in violence. More importantly, the noncruelty that Das discusses also addresses how hijras, though exhibiting a tangential similarity to many forms of exchange, cannot explicate the rules of why they must be given money other than by saying that it is their *haq*. Das writes, "First the quality of noncruelty is demonstrated across species and at moments when it is not through language or through appeals to distant moral concepts as 'obligation' or 'rule-following' but through a sense of togetherness that has developed by the sheer contingency of having been brought together—the fated circumstances of togetherness. Second, that is from within a scene of intimacy that dispositions develop."

It is the togetherness of hijras and the passengers in the Indian social world that allows for an extraction to take place—because when push comes to shove, hijras *can* be violently prevented from collecting their *haq*. The fact that, *in spite* of coercion, they are never refused and their legitimacy is never questioned, is evidence of the social togetherness or intimacy between them and the passengers. This calibration of coercion to avoid violence should be read as adhering to noncruelty rather than rule-following; it is a matter of accountability to others in Spivak's terms rather than one of moral obligation. This is seen most clearly when interactions between hijras and passengers do erupt into brutal physical violence—because even though such violence might resolve the question of whether hijras can or should collect *challa*, it is a resolution that both parties hope to avoid. Their intimacy with the passengers and the laity/polity allows the state to press them into service—press their logic of extraction into service—when it is helpless to achieve a resolution by any less extreme means than through violence.

The being-together that Das invokes is necessarily understood through animals because it brings into relief the "violence that joins life and death," as in "the contemplation on the killing of animals in sacrifice."[40] In this chapter I seek to position hijras as, figuratively, that "animal" that reminds the passengers not only of the violence that is life and death but also, through that animality, of togetherness through which she demands social accountability. Reinvoking one of the interpretive threads of this study, I wish to recall from Chapter 1 the argument that hijras who make their lovers into animals, and from Chapter 2 the argument that they prevent their brothers from becoming one, in the context of the corruption of our times, become animal themselves. In becoming animal, hijras remind us to be accountable to one another socially under the rules of compassion and not under the rules of markets or moral merits.[41]

THE HIJRA POLITICIAN

Another set of newspaper articles completes the picture of togetherness and social intimacy between the polity and hijras, though in this instance not on the trains but in public office. An article entitled "'Incorruptible' Eunuch Takes on Political Giants in Indian Polls," published in 1996, interviews Kali Hijra as she stands for office in the "parliamentary elections as head of the Judicial Reforms Party [JRP]." Kali is quoted as saying, "People believe in what I promise because they know as a eunuch I cannot be lured with wealth, women or sex. They also know we [the JRP] have no religion or gender bias." She clarifies this further: "These leaders have to think of their children when they are out of power and thus they are vulnerable. I am free of all such worries." Several points in this short article merit highlighting, and the relation between them bears explaining. The first is that children make one susceptible to corruption, and consequently being childless frees one from divided loyalties—to either the family or the nation—when those interests are in conflict. "The saree-clad eunuch, who had taken on a female identity said Prime Minister P. V. Narasimha Rao, the father of seven, or Bihar chief minister Laloo Prasad Yadav, the father of nine, are more vulnerable to the temptation of carving out political fiefdoms for their offspring." Hijras like Kali, on the other hand, who has no children of her own to give preferential advantage, wants "to fight for free education for children."[42]

The second point to note is this: while in the first set of articles a hijra's power to shame and to curse with impotence is utilized by the state to force its citizens to pay taxes, in the second set of articles the same power is used to shame the state. An article playing on the word *loktantra,* "democracy," is entitled "Joketantra: The Semiotics of Castration," and reports, "The sexless person in question was effectively used by the electorate to castrate the caste oligarchy which had been running the show all these years." The article astutely points out that it is not just the Dalits, "for whom it is easy to count themselves among the castrated politically speaking," who voted for Shabnam Mausi but the Brahmins as well, "to get better of their rivals, the Rajputs." The author goes on to say that electing a eunuch to the state assembly is "a prank played not so much on democracy—people, after all, did vote—but on the way it is turned into a joke." According to the newspaper article, the voters are expressing their own impotence in convincing the state to fix "bad roads, bad water, bad houses, bad administration, bad money." The author remarks that "the laughter that the eunuch so sadly provokes is double-edged: people are taking a laugh at themselves too, which is where democracy really starts working because it is a question thrown back at its complacent certitudes."[43]

I want to read this laughter of the people as an acknowledgment of the vulnerability of the state, and while recognizing that rules are not being followed, the laughter is also bringing into relief that perhaps rules are too strict to be followed. In these articles, where the politician householder is reiterated as being split between his duties to the state and those to his family, or between *dharma* and *artha,* hijras offer themselves as the ideal candidate to run the state because they do not have a family.[44] Another article reports, "Observers said the tendency to elect Hijras was a sign of voters' frustration with traditional politicians."[45] Kamla Kinnar, a hijra politician, cites her impotence as the basis of her honesty and incorruptibility:

I have no written or ambitious manifesto. Whatever I earned by entertaining people was invested on the welfare of poor, especially for the marriage of 20 girls from impoverished weaver families. Now, I want to raise my voice for addressing the grievances of farmers and weavers whose interests have been destroyed by successive governments. . . . Everybody is working to defeat me, whether it is the UP minister or the jailed sharpshooter. But I am not afraid of either the wealth of the ruling party or the bullets of Sujit Belwa. *Agar is chunav mein meri jaan bhi jaati hai to janta ke liye jayegi.*

The last line, in Hindi, can be translated, "Even if I lose my life in the elections, it will be lost for the public."[46]

Mangesh Bharat Khadye, who ran for the Thane Lok Sabha seat in 2009, "woefully points out that while people overlook the shameful deeds of politicians and parties, a eunuch who talks of protecting the neglected is greeted with smirks and insults."[47] This might be because hijras cannot distance themselves from the political vocabulary that deploys them as symbols of impotence. Hijras might be attempting to translate their impotence into political honesty, but this is not how the public voting one into power is reading her. An article carried by the *New York Times* entitled "Katni Journal: A Pox on Politicians; A Eunuch You Can Trust" reports that persuading Kamla Jaan to run for mayor was "meant as sarcasm, a way to snub the major parties, whose candidates were deemed to be worthless hacks even if of more discernible gender than Ms. Jaan." The article continues, "Reviled, sniggered at and feared as obnoxious and even sorcerous, eunuchs would seem to make unlikely political heroes. But for those who want to express contempt for the political establishment, a eunuch's fallen social rank is a mark in favor." Electing eunuchs seems to be a way that the disenchanted public can attack an ineffective and corrupt state in a nation in which "democracy is seldom practiced within the political parties themselves, where candidacies are doled out as spoils with an eye toward preserving power at the top. Local government is unresponsive to the needs of the people. Elected offices are often thought of as personal property for those foraging for bribes, municipal budgets, always small in a poor country, get squandered, with civic improvements ever outpaced by urban decay."[48]

While the idea of a eunuch heading governmental bodies—free of corruption-inducing family interests—has delicious potential, it seemed the public had not voted for a eunuch because she was beyond dishonesty. For them it was a "mere prank," and they were "tickled by the idea." The article written by Jyotsna Singh for the BBC news service, entitled "Eunuchs Boosted by Voter Disillusion," cites a twenty-six-year-old Ayaz, who says, "They are speaking the truth. Our politicians beg us for votes during elections and don't show up after that. They are not bothered about the people. Why should we vote for them?" The reporter writes, "There may not be many yet who support the eunuchs but a large number of people share the disenchantment pointed out by these eunuchs."[49] While reading these scenes as a staging of the vulnerability of the polity would not be disputed, it needs to be pointed out that the form in which such vulnerability is staged is once again sexual, accenting the impotence of hijras and the corruptibility of the politician stemming from their imperative to reproduce a family. The politicians here are strikingly similar to the *Mahabrahmans* of Parry's ethnography as discussed earlier; it can be argued that in electing hijras, the polity is acknowledging the dilemma of *artha* and *dharma* instead of calling for punitive action against the rulebreakers.

Another article by Parry further complicates this notion of corruption. In "The 'Crisis of Corruption' and the 'Idea of India': A Worm's Eye View," Parry writes, "In some ideal world it may be true that offering a bribe is wrong. But this is not the world that Adhikari sees about him, and he not unreasonably concludes that it is quite unproductive to lose sleep over anything so abstract. . . . At the retail level, at least, giving bribes is doing no more than accommodating oneself to brutal reality." The ethnographic evidence Parry is studying is the widespread participation in corruption by the very same people who complain about its prevalence in the same breath. Parry resolves this contradiction by arguing, "If corruption is the misuse of public office or assets for private interests, then the notion obviously presupposes a clear conceptual separation between the two. In the administration of the Mughal Empire no sharp distinction was drawn. . . . It needed rational legal authority with the idea of public office, impersonal rules and the demarcation of public and private, office and home, to create the discourse of corruption, as we know it."[50] Regardless of one's perception of and complaint about corruption, Parry suggests, one cannot always fight it without dire consequences. What recourse can one take when rules cannot be followed—not only by the other but also by oneself? Das has offered the notion of noncruelty that emerges from togetherness; I want to suggest that the electing of hijra politicians reveals not just the perception of corruption, or the togetherness of hijras and the polity—with the former offering herself as a metaphor for impotence—but the texture of our times when we are hard-pressed to negotiate the violence of the world.

THE FREEDOM OF BONDAGE

Clifford Geertz characterizes the difference between *haq* and *dharma* thus: "If *haqq* negotiates 'is' and 'ought' by construing law as a species of fact, *dharma* does so by construing fact as a species of law, which is very much not the same thing."[51] Geertz's definition of *haq* and its differentiation from *dharma* explains why the state found it logical to unleash hijras upon its constituency and why the public found it fitting to vote for hijra politicians. The mode in which both were extracting what they considered their due from each other—tax, registration, uncorrupted governance—is legitimized because they are reconciling an *ought* with an *is*. The violence that is present in all the scenes associated with hijras, the state, and its people is never questioned precisely because it gains its lawfulness or is a species of the fact that it is the *kalyug*—a time when nothing is as it ought to be.

Before I turn to the myth that hijras have regarding *kalyug*, I want to clarify the relationship between the state and its citizens that is brought to the fore by the way hijras are used in collecting taxes and fighting corruption. This deployment of hijras is possible because of the nature of the interaction that takes place between hijras and the passengers of a train, which I argue is different from begging, and is closer to a form of collecting taxes in view of the threat of violence on the part of both hijras and the passengers. This relationship between the state and its citizens makes sense only when, pace Veena Das, we see citizenship as a "claim rather than a status, which one either has or does not have."[52] Based on this conceptual move— differentiating a claim from a status—Das shows that there is "an underlying allegiance to the idea of preserving life both at the level of the individual and that of the community [which] comes to be expressed in the moment when the State is able to put aside its function to punish infringements of law—thus allowing claims of life to trump claims of law."[53] One can argue that the state reveals the precariousness of its being when it recruits hijras' ability to collect their *haq* from passengers to collect its *haq*—consisting of taxes and information—from its polity. These are moments in which the state is also making a claim on its citizens, and hence one can see the promise in this relationship insofar as the citizens recognize that the state can and does have claims over them. This is a terrible state of affairs, where the state as well as its people are vulnerable vis-à-vis each other but are also dependent on the promise that claims of life or giving somebody one's *haq* will trump the claims of law.

A different way of formulating the relationship of the state with its people, I want to argue, is made visible through the prism of hijras—one that preserves the integrity of the poor, the kind that people Das's ethnography. Merely dilating the notions of precariousness and promise that Das uses would not bring into relief the relationship between the state and its citizens that arises specifically because and through hijras. Rather, I borrow Das's theoretical move by seeing citizenship as a claim rather than a status in order to clarify the relationship between the state and its citizens, both of whom use the impotence of hijras to threaten each other. This move is necessary to understand the threat of impotence that hijras carry, which appears lethal, like a defanged cobra. The difference between status (caste) and claim (citizenship) allows hijras' collection of *haq* once again to be partially similar to caste-based ritual labor that results in economic exchanges in the context of poverty; these exchanges are defined as *jajmani* and are translated as patronage. While hijras can shame the public and their patrons into giving money, sometimes even bordering on extortion, their being is not dependent on caste. This freedom from caste-determined labor is something they earn and enjoy because of the price they pay for their asceticism, their stepping out of kinship and heteronormative reproduction. To this extent hijras perform a critique or remind us of the damages of poverty against the self-sufficiency of hierarchical arrangements of every kind, secular or otherwise.

Georg Simmel wrote that "sociability is, then, the play-form of association and is related to the content-determined concreteness of association as art is related to reality." This sociability, play-form, or "social game" is necessary because it calibrates the claims that the individual and the social can make on each other. Simmel continues:

Sociability is the play-form also for the ethical forces of concrete society. The great problems placed before these forces are that the individual has to fit himself into a whole system and live for it: that, however, out of this system values and enhancement must flow back to him, that the life of the individual is but a means for the ends of the whole, the life of the whole but an instrument for the purposes of the individual. Sociability carries the seriousness, indeed the frequent tragedy of these requirements, over into its shadow world, in which there is no friction, because shadows cannot impinge upon one another.[54]

If sociability is a play-form that calibrates the individual to the social and vice versa so as to help prevent the tragedy of such compromises; if it is what Simmel later calls "the freedom of bondage," then I suggest that what takes place between hijras and the passengers, and by extension between the state and its citizens, is a play that averts the tragedy of claims that citizens and state make on each other, preserving what Das (citing Didier Fassin) identifies as the "politics of life." While both the citizen and the state have other options to extract their claims, their *haq*—for example, a revolution on the part of the citizens or imprisonment on the part of the state—they use instead hijras, who can infect one with impotence and shame—but not really. They are like defanged cobras that look poisonous and appear lethal but—like Simmel's shadows—truly are not. I argue that what is implied by this mode of extracting claims is a politics of life as well, insofar as it forestalls the tragedies that are often the consequence of extracting claims. The scene of collecting *challa* on trains that serves as an allegory of claiming *haq* prophesies the physical violence that can erupt between the state and its citizens. We must read Das's conceptual move in seeing citizenship as a claim rather than a status as an addendum to Simmel's definition of sociability as a play-form; when one is playing a game there is a certain set of claims that we make on the other players—to follow certain rules—which in this case is to try to preserve life in the *kalyug*.

KALYUG

Before I analyze hijras' myth of the *kalyug*, a brief description of South Asian chronology by Romila Thapar will be helpful to set the scene:

Each major time cycle, *mahayuga* or great cycle, also referred to as the *caturyuga* of four cycles, is divided into four cycles, the *yugas*—Krta (or Satya), Dvapara, Treta and Kali—the names derived from the numbers at the throw of dice from the highest to the lowest and therefore carrying the suggestion of fate implicit in time. The condition of man and the world has changed from the earliest times which were utopian to the ultimate decline in the fourth *yuga*, the *kali-yuga*, which is the current cycle.[55]

We must begin with Thapar's delicate suggestion that the current age, the *kali-yuga* or *kalyug*, is when the throw of dice or the chances are against us. The reason for such bad luck is that, as *The Law Code of Manu* (*Manusmriti*) states, "There is one set of laws for men in the Krta Age, another in the Treta, still another in the Dvapara, and a different set in the Kali, in keeping with the progressive shortening taking place in each Age. Ascetic toil, they say, is supreme in the Krta Age, knowledge in the Treta, sacrifice in Dvapara, and gift-giving alone in Kali."[56] We are coming closer to an understanding of exchange in our current day and age. Neither asceticism, nor knowledge, nor even sacrifice is enough to strengthen our chances to survive these times. "In the Krta Age, the Law is whole, possessing all four feet; and so is truth. People never acquire any property through unlawful means. By acquiring such property, however, the Law is stripped of one foot in each of the subsequent Ages; through theft, falsehood, and fraud, the Law disappears a foot at a time."[57]

What Patrick Olivelle has translated as law is *dharma*, which can be defined alternatively as the proper rules of conduct. *Dharma* is represented as a bull, which helps to illuminate why the image of our time, the *kalyug*, is a bull without any legs to stand on. The book of Manu further states, "Krta-age, Treta-age, Dvapara-age, and Kali-age—the king's activities constitute all these; for the king is said to be the age. When he is asleep, he is Kali; when he is awake, he is Dvapara; when he is ready to undertake operations, he is Treta and when he is on the march, he is Krta."[58] The unchecked corruption that defines our age is seen allegorically through the image of the king who is sleeping, unaware of the injustices taking place in his realm. Dharma, or law, is incapable of checking anybody, having lost his legs, and only gift-giving reigns supreme, more effective than asceticism, knowledge, and sacrifice. Here lies the difference between *haq* and *dharma* as noted by Geertz, which Das clarifies. The rules of *dharma*, according to Das's reading of *appadharma*, can be suspended and substituted with another set during times of distress, thereby rendering some claims or *haq* viable that at another time would not have existed.

Now, let us look at the myth of *kalyug* widely cited and recited by hijras. In this myth Rama, the seventh avatar of Vishnu, was ordered by his father, King Dasharatha, to relinquish his right to the throne and undertake an exile in the forest for fourteen years because of the plotting of his father's other wife. When he left to go to the forest, the whole kingdom came to see him off; they were weeping with sorrow at his departure. At the edge of the forest he commanded all the men and women to return to their homes and resume their daily lives. Since he had not told hijras what to do, they remained there for fourteen years awaiting his return. When Rama returned, he was amazed to see them and asked why they had not gone back. Hijras replied that Rama had just addressed the men and women and did not say anything about or to hijras. Rama was very moved by their faith and granted them the boon that during *kalyug*, hijras would rule the earth.[59]

This myth was recited to me as well one night in Bhawanipatna, when Damru, Nandita, and I were strolling around and four men driving by in a car stopped. One of the men asked Damru and Nandita to come with him next week to another district headquarters town, and they agreed. Once the men drove off, I inquired who they were and what they wanted; Damru said these men worked for the local Member of the Legislative Assembly, and whenever his party members went to give speeches in various villages, he would take hijras with them. Hijras were asked to show up and testify to the people that these party politicians are not corrupt and that hijras support them. Everyone trusts the word of a hijra because she doesn't have any reason to be corrupt, Damru continued—thus reiterating hijras as a figure that cannot be corrupted.

A newspaper article that appeared in the year 2000 bearing the title "The Kalyug Rulers" evokes this myth in the course of reporting on Asha Devi, an ex-MLA hijra from Gorakhpur. It reads, "If nothing else, Devi has the scriptures backing her claim. Lord Rama had prophesied that eunuchs would rule once Kalyug descended on earth. It officially arrived in February this year when Shabnam Mausi won a seat from Sohagpur constituency in Madhya Pradesh as an independent candidate. With Asha Devi, Kalyug seems to be truly upon us."[60]

Yet one more definition of *kalyug*, this time from the *Mahabharata*, will help lead this account to conclusion. The third book of the *Mahabharata*, entitled the *Vana Parva*, has for its content a conversation between the great king Yudhisthra and the great sage Markandeya. Yudhishtra requests to hear Markandeya's "account with the causes of everything." Markandeya, in describing the *kalyug*, says to Yudhishtra, "Householders, out of fear of the burden of taxes, will become thieves, and others hiding under the guise of hermits will live off trade." Markandeya continues, "The Brahmins will become like crows. . . . As they are oppressed by the Dasyus and are constantly oppressed by evil kings with the burden of taxes; and giving up their poise."[61] This version of the *kalyug* would fit very well with the fact that the citizens of the state feel the need to escape paying taxes and part with their money only when threatened with shame or impotence. This closely parallels the unquestioning manner with which passengers give up their hard-earned money to hijras when they come aboard the trains.

Unfortunately, hijras are not incorruptible. Even a brief glance in the news archive disproves this claim. They do not shy away from injuring passengers, as the aforementioned ethnographic scenes have demonstrated; nor do they shy away from injuring railway officials when asked for railway tickets.[62] A telling newspaper article entitled "Eunuch among Five Arrested for Murder" informs us that "a eunuch and her four friends were arrested for murdering and robbing her 'godfathers' in Himachal Pradesh two years ago, police said Friday." The article cites a police officer as claiming, "Asha was in a live-in with Babloo. She frequently visited her godfathers with her colleagues, and tempted by their wealth one day decided to rob them." The official continues, "Afraid that she would be identified, Chaudhary and Khan slit the throat of the victims and the gang fled from the spot." Another newspaper article entitled "Eunuch Held for Killing Live-In Partner" has the police inform the reporter, "A eunuch was arrested here [in New Delhi] on Saturday for killing her live-in partner in a fit of rage." The police continue, "Nisha used to help him financially, Nisha also helped him in setting up a shop at Sona Vihar and used to spend money on him. . . . Two years ago Nisha came in contact with Hasmukh and started living with him. Hasmukh too exploited her and extorted money from her." The article quotes the police: "Frustrated with Hasmukh, she deserted him and came back to Surender. . . . After buying a car and bike with Nisha's money Surender was pressing her to buy a house. Surender also stole Nisha's Rs. 3.5 Lakh. . . . When she asked for the money Surender hit her. Unable to bear the humiliation, Nisha hit him on the head and stabbed him to death."[63] Yet another newspaper article, "Eunuch Gang Leader Killed in Encounter with Noida Police," reports, "Atique, a leader of a eunuch gang in Ghaziabad, was wanted in more than a dozen cases. He came to the limelight after he was made the prime accused in the murder of a Eunuch from a rival gang."[64]

Hijras are not different from Parry's priests, who are constrained by the real world to retain the money they receive, hence are unable to augment the amount they give back as *dana*. Newspaper articles such as one entitled "2 Eunuchs Found Killed, Jewellery and Cash Missing" inform us that "Vimlesh owned the three-storey residential complex and four cars." The article goes on to suggest that Vimlesh's adopted son and her driver, who had been missing with one of her cars, might have killed the two hijras. The investigation yielded the following: "It has been reported that Vimlesh and Khalil had some sort of physical relationship. But that changed when Sultan reportedly became the new companion of Vimlesh."[65] Another article headlined, "Eunuchs Robbed of Rs 50 Lakhs" informs us that "around a dozen masked robbers targeted a 'dera' of eunuchs in Kalka during the intervening night of Tuesday and Wednesday and made away with Rs 50 Lakh in cash and jewellery including 800g gold."[66] These news articles suggest that hijras do not escape the constraints of the real world; their money, like that of the Brahmin priests of Parry's ethnography, is also tainted. Against the grain of Damru's narrative that hijras are the *saccha fakirs*, authentic fakirs (mendicants or ascetics), there are plenty of instances of hijras stealing money and possessions from their clients when their trousers are down.

How are we then to make sense of the myth that hijras will rule the earth during *kalyug*? Hijra politicians, the election of whom is cited as evidence that this prophecy is coming true, argue against the notion that the public elected them as a joke to undermine the authority of the state and to shame the corrupt, impotent government. They claim, rather, that the public elected them because hijras cannot be corrupted. Hijras do rule the earth during our current time of the *kalyug*, I would suggest, but not in the way these hijra politicians argue. If the current government is beleaguered in face of a thieving public that shames them and equates them with hijras to mark their impotence, then we must expand the category *hijra* to encompass the government as well. The public that is oppressed by the burden of taxes and is impotent in the face of evil kings in this time—when *dharma* is standing on its last leg—must likewise be enfolded into the category *hijra*. Both the state and the public align themselves with hijras when facing each other. Everyone is a hijra. As the mythic sage Markandeya warned, everybody will be equal to the Sudras [the lowest caste]. Hijras, rather than being incorruptible, exemplify the corruption of the world. Their promises, like those of the politicians, are empty; they collect and hoard money that, like the money of the priests, cannot fructify but instead brings about their death. They endorse politicians for money and sell for a price their reputation of being authentic ascetics who have only the best interests of the public at heart.

Das has argued that "the relation between the other *yugas* and Kaliyuga, then, is that of the conceptual order to the empirical order."[67] Instead of being estranged from the state, hijras' role in social life reflects the politics of our time, when there is corruption or a perception of corruption both in the state's bureaucracy and among the citizenry. Hijras emerge as a figure that lubricates this acrimonious relationship. Like a defanged cobra, hijras threaten with a virtual bite. The appearance of the threat, in Simmel's words, carries the seriousness and the tragic consequences of the social into a shadow world and thereby attenuates it. That such deception can sometimes be worse than the violence it seeks to prevent or contain exhibits in itself the quality of *kalyug*, when things are not what they seem and there are no grounds on which one can know the correct rules of conduct.[68] During such times, we cannot but yield to the debts and liabilities of compassion.

4

LOVE MAY TRANSFORM ME

When I first came to do fieldwork, there was a spat going on between two of my informants, Jaina and Azgari. Their shops were on the same street, with a couple shops separating them. Jaina refused to come to Azgari's shop and have tea with her. When I asked her why, she replied, "Ask her. So much trouble has been created over one boy." The trouble as it was told to me unfolded in bits and pieces over a month. A young boy had moved to Bhadrak a year ago and had struck up an amorous friendship with Azgari.[1] The boy known as Bablu (usually just referred to as Khalifa's grandson) would always be found at Azgari's shop, and they would often buy each other sweets: Azgari would give him money to eat some snacks and Bablu would buy Azgari tea and paan. Azgari had a longstanding festering feud with Bablu's father's young brother. They both used to collect money for the annual cricket tournament that would take place in the village, but Azgari had complained that the man would never do the work he was hired to do but would show up for the feast at the end of the tournament; she eventually got him kicked off the committee. This had obviously not gone down very well with Bablu's uncle. Once, Bablu had a fight with some of the boys and had run away and hidden in Azgari's shop in the evening. Later, in the night, when Azgari was wrapping up her day, bathing at the nearby tube well, his family came out looking for him; she told them she had no idea where Bablu was, even though she had seen him slip inside her shop. When Bablu appeared again in the morning, the carpenter across the street from Azgari's shop informed the uncle that he had seen Bablu come out of Azgari's shop in the morning.

The uncle then complained to other people that Azgari had "spoilt the boy" (*bigaar diya*) and that he should be taught a lesson. A *panchayat* (village council) was called during which the uncle asked his nephew whether he had spent the night with Azgari; the boy lied and said "no." He was asked whether he had ever "done it" with Azgari (*uske saath kiya hai ki nahin*), and he again replied "no." A little more must be said about how Bablu came to be with Azgari in the first place. Bablu was living with his mother's family in another place before he was moved back to his father's place in Shankarpur, Bhadrak. His father had asked Azgari to keep an eye on him and to teach him the cycle-repair trade if the boy showed any interest. During the *panchayat* the uncle started beating the boy mercilessly and asked him to tell the truth, but the boy kept on denying that he had spent the night or "done it" with Azgari. People stopped the uncle and said, "If you beat him like this, of course he will say yes." Azgari said, "Then I told the uncle that if he has a doubt, both of us should go to the *mazar* and take an oath; whoever is lying would fall ill on the fifteenth day. The uncle then refused to do this. I was saved because I would have had to take a false oath and would have fallen ill." People disbanded and the hullabaloo died down, but the boy kept on coming to the shop. After a week of my being there, Azgari came to me and said, "I have told him to not come to my shop anymore." I asked her, "Why?" and she replied, "Because when he used to sit there, he would touch me, pinch me, tease me, people would see, and after all the fuss they would start thinking that perhaps something is going on here, so I told him not to come here anymore."

After another week or two Azgari came to my room late in the night and said in a tired melancholic voice, "What did they get from creating so much trouble? So what if he was sitting at my shop and teasing me and pinching me and he bought me some small things like tea and snacks—how was it harming anybody? If I take a small vessel of water from an ocean, is the ocean poorer?" I looked visibly confused at this metaphor—was the youth an ocean of love?—but I didn't say anything. Azgari noted the confusion and tried to explain it by starting to say, "A man is like an ocean . . ." but then looked confused herself and ambled away into the night. After a few weeks, Azgari came again to my room in the middle of the night with some paan and a cup of tea. She told me a story that clarified the metaphor she had used:

Once, a long time ago, a pir was asked by God to leave India and travel somewhere else to preach Islam. After traveling for days, months, and years he settled on a place, but that land was owned by a very rich Jewish man. He asked his followers to bring him a small vessel of water so that he could wash himself and begin his prayers. His followers went to the lake but the Jewish man who had heard that this preacher had come to his land had ordered his soldiers to prevent the men from collecting water. The followers went back to the preacher and the preacher himself came to the lake and asked for permission to collect some water. After hearing the soldiers deny him, the entire lake itself came to the shore and poured itself into the small vessel.

Here I wish to argue that Azgari, through her invocation, "A man is like an ocean," was using a mythical reference to signal a certain understanding of sex and consent.[2] The folktale of the pir with his magical powers is effectively linked with her own affair with the young boy, and the boy's consent to the sexual encounter is made apparent by the parallel drawn between him and the water of the lake: just as the water comes willingly into the pir's small vessel because of the pir's powers and his proximity to God—making the impossible possible—so the boy came willingly to Azgari, testifying to the truth and purity of her love.

PEDAGOGY, PLAY, AND CONSENT

To understand the issue of consent at stake here we must also understand how the politics of penetration complicate it. The phrase *bigaar diya* signals something other than consensual or nonconsensual sex. Literally it means *to spoil*; for example, spoilt children are called *bigda hua*, and to spoil someone's well-laid plans would be described as *kaam bigadna*. With all these semantic possibilities in mind, the accusation leveled at Azgari makes more sense. First of all, she was not accused of raping the young man; rape was thought of narrowly as penetration in Bhadrak and furthermore was limited to the rape of women. Stories and details about young college-going girls being raped was often told, for example, and men jilted in love often threatened to rape the women who were either being coy and playing hard to get or just not interested in them. The accusation of *bigarna* connotes impropriety—the unmarried youth is not being taught how to live and organize his life in a manner deemed fruitful/proper/profitable. Lawrence Cohen has written how anal sex in India is organized along the axis of the *gaandu* and the *londebaaz*, the one who gets fucked and the one who "takes pleasure in young men," or pederasty, a pastime/hobby for royals and the rich (*nawabi shauk*).[3] This *nawabi* pleasure of fucking aligns itself with the sexual metaphors of feudalism and its various and variegated reiterations in modern India.

Let us make the connection between the pleasures of fucking for the *londebaaz* and the crises of economy that it implies.[4] Ruth Vanita, in her introduction to her indispensable work of translation of Pandey Bechan Sharma's *Chocolate and Other Writings on Male Homoeroticism*, writes, "The word *chocolate*, which Ugra [Bechan Sharma's nom de plume], in his foreword, claimed to have invented as a synonym for the popular term *laundebaazi* (boy chasing), rapidly came to be used by everyone in the debate, including supporters and opponents of Ugra. Today this connotation of the word is no longer widely known, but from the mid-1920s to the mid-1930s, it functioned in the Hindi literary world as a convenient code word that enabled avoidance of more explicit language."[5] Vanita herself offers a few explanations underlining the logic behind this code: "Given the long Indian tradition of celebrating the virtues of milk products, such as ghee, butter, and cream, the popularity of chocolate in India is not surprising," and she remarks on "how ineradicable Western tastes are part of modern Indian identity." She speculates, "Chocolate is one of the most widely amiable consumer items in India; it is so indigenized that its name has become a Hindi word, yet it is non-Indian in origin, compared to Indian sweetmeats like laddoos. . . . It suggests that an attempt to eradicate homosexuality in modern India would be as self-defeating and anti-pleasure as an attempt to eradicate the taste for chocolate." Interestingly, after stating that "the connotation of the word is no longer widely known," she records a comment by a "woman activist who works with a sexuality rights organization." The woman, on hearing her present an earlier version of the essay, remarked that *chocolate* is still used as street lingo among some groups of non-English-speaking homosexual males to refer to an attractive effeminate man or boy.[6]

Though none of the stories mentions explicitly whether chocolates are the ones fucking or fucked, the depiction of the sex between the chocolate and the man either assumes the reader's knowledge or is communicated through ellipsis; the narration concerning the youth is always coded in a way that renders him penetrated. For example, the penetrator takes on the role of half-crazed male protagonists of legendary love stories: "He admitted to the Thakur at the start that such love becomes infernal when it grows impure and perverted by desire. So at the outset he would gaze upon him from a distance and consider himself the equivalent of Majnun and Farhad." The youth, by contrast, is cast in the female roles of legendary lovers or prostitutes, and within the narrative logic acts with the coquetry of a courtesan: "Gradually the rustic boy's face began to lose its beauty. Its boyish innocence and tenderness began to be replaced by a prostitute's shamelessness and harshness."[7] We never hear in the short stories the voice of the youth, as is to be expected since, as Lawrence Cohen has shown elsewhere, in this world of *karna* and *karwana*—of doing and being done to, of fucking and being fucked—the pleasures are taken by feudal landlords in exploitation, and there is no depiction or form given to the pleasures of being penetrated; it remains abject, beyond description.[8]

Though Vanita does not remark on the politics of penetration in these stories, committing instead to a formalist reading of the text that prevents an easy reading of the stories as purely moralistic or didactic, thus recuperating the political purposes of translating them in the first place, there is nonetheless a discernible economy of being fucked and fucking present. While the *laundebaaz*, the penetrator, upon discovery of his *shauk* or love faces public shame, calumny, excommunication, and imprisonment, the beloved or the chocolate, the penetrated, either dies of tuberculosis caused by homosexuality, more specifically by being fucked, or is let go narratively and figuratively with a mild punishment.[9] The implication here is that no one would want to be fucked; youths and chocolates have been seduced and become wayward—they have become spoilt, if you will—and can be made to see the light and follow the right path. The *laundebaaz* in these stories are the ones with inflated agency, in view of their age, and are immoral, given the way they use their privilege to seduce.

One of the characters, whose eccentricity undermines his strict moral preachings, as Vanita notes, says:

O beautiful young men! You do not yet know what this world is like. You are filled with enthusiasm and curiosity. You do not know the difference between good and bad. That is why I say to you, Do not consider my words a joke. This is not the age to learn bad things. You should not play the drama of love now; do not get seduced and hide your face on any-one's chest. Refrain from understanding the mysteries of embraces and kisses. Don't sell your beautiful bodies, your blossoming cheeks, your red lips! . . . Otherwise, once this beauty is destroyed, this dazzling face is blackened, the redness of these fair lips dries up, the shyness of these eyes dies, you will face nothing but hatred and disgust in the world. . . . As soon as nature or men steal these from you, you will become three a penny. . . . Don't let any man kiss your lips, don't let any intoxicated one stroke your cheeks, don't let any demon press your tender chest to his iron heart! You are not sex objects. You are men, you are gods, you are God.[10]

While the fucker gets off with discipline and punishment, the fucked is either seen not to have the desire to be penetrated, or, when he does, he dies of tuberculosis or has the beauty of his face replaced by a "prostitute's shame-lessness and harshness."[11] Lawrence Cohen offers a touching ethnographic snippet of a man who sketches his penis on a card to give his beloved, thereby forcing the anthropologist to locate the grammar of love, sex, and penetra-tions that go against depictions of sodomitical violence.[12] I mention this blink-and-miss portion of Cohen's iconoclastic essay because it argues against the immorality of Bechan Sharma's *laundebaazi*. We have yet to ac-count for the ethnographic scene involving Azgari and the boy who opened this chapter, in which no feudality existed that could be aligned with being fucked, either in age, since Khalifa's grandson was much, much younger than Azgari and was penetrating a hijra rather than being penetrated by a feudal lord, or because of financial standing—his family was neither richer nor poorer than Azgari. The fact that the youth was penetrating and was not being penetrated implies this was not the *bigaarna* or spoiling of the kind that the *laundebaaz* or the fucker effects, but a different *bigaarna*. It was something that, I suspect, would not have resulted in such a ruckus had Azgari not picked a fight with the boy's uncle, or had the carpenter not in-formed him.

I am going to take a detour not only because I want to offer a different reading of chocolate, pedagogy, penetration, consent, and coercion than the one mentioned previously, but also because it will help us complete the se-miotic field of penetration that folds against itself when age is thrown into the equations of *londebaazi*, *karna*, and *karwana*. Azgari had been repairing cycles for years and had taught several boys the practices of the trade; they were now repairing bicycles all around Bhadrak, and this was one of the reasons Azgari was much loved and respected in the town. When she was swamped with customers, she would send them to her former apprentices and would also receive customers from them. She was giving me a history of all the boys who had passed through her hands and how her generosity prevented her from becoming an easy target for bullying or harassment. She used to say, "People know if they say something or do something, all my boys will come armed to save me." I asked her where she had learned her trade, and she grinned and amusedly told me the story of her master. "I was very young when I started working in a shop near Charampa. He was a big man, a pathan; whenever I used to make a mistake, he used to fuck me. For years it went on like this, if there was ever a mistake he used to first fuck me, then tell me how to do it correctly. Oh, he was big *karnewala*; he also used to take good care of me, feed me, and give me money and chocolates, chai, and other things to eat. Then, when I turned sixteen or seventeen, he helped me to start my own shop."

Earlier ethnographies are replete with narratives of *bigarna* and *bigaarna*. Vyas and Shingala's *The Life Style of the Eunuchs* records the following: "While interviewing them, one explained that he was the schoolboy from a well-reputed family, his teacher used to call the students at his place for teaching purpose. The teacher was not charging the fees. But exposed him toward unnatural sexual relationship. The boy become habituated and used to act as a female. People used to laugh at him for his behavior. And it was unmanageable and uncontrollable for him to live. He met this people and became a eunuch." Yet another hijra tells the authors, "Saheb, how little you know the world. A damned sodomite in the chawl in which I lived misused me even before I had grown a moustache. He buggered me by force and often. After a while I began liking it too. When I was twenty-one, I was glad to get myself castrated."[13] These stories might seem to cohere with simplistic notions of desire, pleasure, and violence—and with the moralistic notions of *bigarna* that Ugra warns us about—but when Gayatri Reddy probes more deeply, these narratives begin to lose traction. Hijras in her ethnography tell her, "From birth, I always liked to put *moggus* [rice-flour designs drawn on the ground, typically by women], play with girls, and help with the cooking and cleaning. I liked only men and was spoiled by them early in life. I used to make up games where I was the wife and this boy I liked was my husband, and I would make him spoil me."[14] She writes, "The extraordinary violence that each of them suffered appeared almost ubiquitous in all their lives. Several koti narratives would date their entry into 'this line' from the point in their lives when they were 'spoiled' by their friend, neighbors, and teachers."[15] Suresh, a koti, told Reddy, "I entered this line first when I was 'raped' by my teacher in school. I was nine or ten years old, and my teacher told me that he wanted to talk to me after class. Then he 'raped' me. I didn't know anything at that time about 'homosex,' or kotis, or anything. I didn't enjoy it at all that time, but slowly, slowly I began to enjoy, and now I am a 'homosex.'"[16]

Yet another vignette in Reddy's ethnography, recounted by Vikas, goes as follows: "I still remember the day he came to our village. . . . It was a Saturday. We did not have school on that day and so I was playing in the garden. I saw this man on the road. He was wearing a very smart uniform and he looked so handsome, I cannot tell you! He looked at me straight, and my heart was going *dhud-dhud*." Over the next couple of years, as Vikas grew to late adolescence, the navy serviceman and he "became good friends." One day his friend invited Vikas into his house and "spoiled" him. He then quickly added, "I should not say that I did not enjoy. I also enjoyed. But once you enjoy like that, once you enjoy 'homosex,' you cannot go back."[17] Reddy analyzes the notion of spoiling and writes:

> The "spoiling" (*cedu* or *cedugottu* in Telugu) referred to the sexual experiences of many hijras and other kotis when they were either receptive partners in their sexual relationships with men or, as they indicated in a few instances, "raped" by them. Most of these kotis said they were "spoiled" by these men *because* they were kotis, that is, they actively desired receptive, anal intercourse, and the men they had sex with knew kotis enjoyed their sexual practice. Others, however, said that it was this first sexual experience that "spoiled" them for future penetrative/heterosexual intercourse, "weakening [their] organ" and subsequently making them either impotent or able to "enjoy only 'homosex.'" Whatever their causal attribution, as they categorically state, "Now [we] are kotis and there is nothing [we] can do about it."[18]

The cause of the spoiling, notwithstanding the violence of first sexual encounters, is conflated with the result of the spoiling in these narratives, making clear the irony in Ugra's moralistic tales. The penetration did not result in spoiling; hijras find it necessary to tell Reddy that they were already kotis, and they would make the men "spoil" them. The biological gloss given by them regarding their impotence, which they claim makes them enjoy homosex, is undermined by the disgust they feel toward hijras and kotis who are married and have children. Clearly, then, even if penetration causes impotence, it doesn't necessarily result in making them into kotis or hijras. Reddy writes:

> In one case, however, I was explicitly asked to intervene by "talking sense into" one koti (BR), who had abandoned his wife and children and temporarily joined the hijras. The other kotis—BR's friends—told me to try to get BR to "live a decent life and go back to his wife." It was significant that only after BR joined the hijras was he believed to be leading an indecent life. Prior to this, he had been cruising the park with his other koti friends for at least ten years. Even though he had been married all this time, the koti lifestyle was not considered transgressive in the same way as his current (proto) hijra lifestyle.[19]

We have reached an odd place: Spoiling through penetration doesn't make young people of various ages into hijras or kotis; rather, they were spoilt, they claim, because they were kotis (broadly taken to refer to those who are effeminate and get penetrated). Some of them say they became impotent because they were spoilt. Fair enough, but that did not make them into hijras or kotis, because impotence is not the only reason for becoming a hijra—as hijras and kotis who are married to women and have children testify. The only thing that is common to all these narratives of becoming hijra is the pleasure in homosex or in being penetrated; even the ones who are married want to leave their wives and kids and be fucked. Sometimes the pleasure is refracted in narratives and traced from the first glance—a glance that makes the heart go *dhud-dhud*—through repeated fucking to the moment when they can't enjoy anything else besides being fucked. The spoiling then refers to the transformation of the violence of penetration into the pleasures of being penetrated.

Leo Bersani, in his article *Pedagogy and Pederasty*, writes, "[The penetrated boy in a pederastic relationship] will be worthy of becoming a free adult Greek male citizen only if, while accepting the desires of the pursuant man, he manages not to share any sensations with him—that is, to experience any sexual pleasure. A kind of sublimation of sexuality is apparently possible within the sexual act itself: it is by mastering the pleasure of passivity in a situation in which he is defined *as* passivity that the boy lays the foundation for the spiritualizing transformation of sex into the socially acceptable relation of *philia*, or friendship."[20] Penetration is never or rather shouldn't be pleasurable for the boy, and it is pleasurable for the man only to the extent that he discovers that it is truth that he loves through boys. Hijras in their narratives resist sublimation and are failed subjects— politically and in every other way. This would hardly be news if Bersani had not rescued failure by reading Foucault against himself, writing, "The writer's resistance to his culture can lie—as Foucault had abundantly shown in his earlier work—not in the factitious power of a mind mythically exercised into a kind of self-divestiture, but rather in the excessive passivity of his surrender to the coercive seductions of what he 'silently thinks.'"[21] Azgari and all the other hijras, in resisting sublimation and surrendering to the pleasures of coercive seductions, are failures; but there are also some resistances to such failure that bring us closer to understanding the "spoiling" that Azgari was doing in being penetrated rather than penetrating.

STAYING WEIRD

Michael Moon, in his monograph on Henry Darger, constructs an argument that veers away from interpreting Darger's paintings as symptomatic of his personal history or fantasies of sexual violence. He argues that far from being strange depictions of extraordinary violence, and given the history of the figure of the child in the Christian cosmos of the West, Darger "took on the role of witness to the terrible ordinariness of violence in the history of the twentieth century—especially violence against children, and specifically against girls."[22] Moon reconstructs the milieu of the early twentieth century in which orphans like Darger grew up through the literature that was found in Darger's room and the various pulp fictions that Darger "plagiarized" to create his own magnum opus and juxtaposes it against the other literatures of fantasies—or fantasies of literature that are well known, notably the ones written by the Brontë children but carried onto adulthood by Branwell Brontë. He writes, "I understand both Branwell Brontë's and Henry Darger's apparent (and shared) predilection for scenes of gruesome and grotesque mortality as the strong desire they also shared to expose and explore what they perceived as the rottenness of the rule of cosmic law in their respective worlds."[23] Moon concludes by arguing that "the almost intolerable truth that makes both their bodies of work still such unwelcome—and indeed in most ways unreceived—'news' is that the rottenness of much of what they have to show us may be neither an effect nor a symptom of their personal histories or psychologies, but a fundamental and constitutive element of their—and our—worlds."[24]

The rule of cosmic law whose rottenness and ungrounded and ungroundable foulness that Azgari exposed was that which governed the economy of semen. As I mentioned in the introduction, much has been written about semen and its resultant contradictions in South Asia. Veena Das writes, "The man in his young adulthood faces a peculiar contradiction whereby abstaining from sex is considered to bestow great power and good health and yet satisfaction of instinctual urges is also considered necessary."[25] Lawrence Cohen has extended this argument to show the inevitable failure of economy that is implicit in the inheritance of this contradiction, which is recognized metonymically through the much-discussed anxiety of semen-loss syndrome. In short, he argues that even though there is much emphasis on semen retention and its preciousness valorized in many texts and contexts, the rules of exchange that are prescribed can hardly be followed—not even gods can adhere to them; it would be like outdoing the atom bomb. In fact, "the conservative logic of accumulation makes possible the expensive play of semen, its prodigious and potlatch exchange, its passionate waste."[26] The fact that life is lived against the grain and rules are broken was obvious to the people of Cohen's ethnography as well as to the good people of Bhadrak and was probably the reason Azgari's affair with the boy did not create a moral dilemma or lead to outrage for the villagers. They did not beat Azgari up or take her to the police station, but it still provided enough ground for the boy's uncle to use it as an excuse to address other grievances and grudges.

To understand what Bersani, pace Foucault, calls the resistances of failure and how Cohen has read hijra bodies as an "utterly abject yet indestructible and ultimately triumphant body," we must understand the way in which the rotten law that governs the exchange of semen is subverted by hijras.[27] The various contradictions in the rules of semen exchange that have been recorded by Cohen were present and talked about in Bhadrak, as well. Youths would often retort to hijras, teasing them: "My parents spend so much money to feed me so that my power increases; why are you making me waste it?" They would often come up to hijras and me to ask in a whisper what they can do about their "nightfall" (nocturnal emissions/wet dreams). Jaina would naughtily reply, "If you don't give it to us, then this is what will happen." But these are the boys who did come to hijras to fuck them. It is because, on the one hand, while they received a lot of care and attention from their families, and their "power" increased with the sacrifices made by their families to feed them, on the other hand they realized that their semen lost its value very soon if it could not be converted to money. Thus, one way in which the semen of the young men regained value and power was through being desired by hijras.

The Osellas, who have studied masculinities in Kerala for decades, write, "For boys in the poorest laboring families, adolescence hardly exists: they move from an impoverished and deprived childhood in which their parents are unable to protect them from the knowledge of adult realities into a young manhood, which immediately demands that they take their share of responsibility by dealing with those realities."[28] The Osellas' ethnography offers several heartbreaking portraits of young men with bleak prospects who have their bodies, beauty, and youth robbed in backbreaking labor in the cities and who return home defeated and broken.[29] But youths did not need to leave Bhadrak to learn the hard lessons of life; their lives would change overnight, and they would be expected to tackle the world with the odds against them without any warning. In the mornings Jaina and I used to have our breakfast sitting in a small shack where an old couple would sell cooked food. Incidentally, their only son had died in Calcutta some years before in an accident at a construction site where he worked. An old woman used to have her breakfast there as well; I had noticed her before but never paid her any attention. One such day, a boy somewhere around twelve, if not younger, got off his cycle and asked her to give him some food. She refused. The boy turned to the old shopkeeper, who was frying some puris, and asked him to give him some food. The old woman forbade the old shopkeeper to give him any: "If you give him food, I am not paying for it, you can give it out of your own wish." The boy got a bit belligerent and screamed, "Give me some food, I haven't eaten the whole day." The old woman did not say anything and continued eating. I looked at Jaina and gestured with my eyebrows; she piped up to the boy, who was muttering to himself angrily as he was leaving, "Oh, come, I'll give you some food," but the boy was already cycling away furiously, crying. Jaina chuckled, and the old woman turned to us and said, "No, there is no need, don't spoil him; if he is so hungry, he will find a way to earn money" (*bhuk lagega to apne aap paisa kamana seekh jayega*). She paid and left, and I remember thinking how cruel the old woman was. Jaina probably read my thoughts, chuckled, and said, "Oh, this old woman turned out to be a big fucker, she will fuck everybody" (*oh, yeh budiya to bahut bari chodhnewali nikli, sab ko chodh ke rak degi*).

The instance of spoiling that the grandmother was warning against put in danger the capacity of the boy to earn money for food; he would not learn to work hard to feed an empty stomach. I want to argue that Azgari, in getting fucked by the youth Bablu, spoilt him in a similar way. The spoiling Azgari offered put in danger the value of semen, so precious, being dispensed so luxuriously in a hijra. The sex with hijras became important because it shored masculinity when the chances of meeting the backbreaking expectations for young men in rural Odisha are slim, and it strips one of health, youth, and flesh. Fucking luxuriously is where expectations are met, success tasted. The family, as the Osellas have noted, forces the poor youth to become a man; his semen, which is constructed as a synecdoche for his masculinity and the value of his body, is expected to result in him earning money and supporting the family. The family expects the sacrifices made by them to increase the semen, the power of the youth, to yield some returns. Unfortunately, young boys often discovered that the world is not that invested in them; they are dispensable, and the odds are stacked against the illiterate young men of Bhadrak. Becoming a householder, a husband, and a father would have reinscribed the potency and value to their semen. In fact, as the Osellas have noted, marriage was an important rite of passage for nonbrahmanical youths in becoming a man. Though sought after, however, marriage was often out of reach for the young men in Bhadrak, given that parents often desired to get their daughters married to employed young men who were financially stable, even if it meant that the girl's conjugal house would be elsewhere. During my fieldwork, people in the village would often deliberate on the dangers of having their daughters married off to Arabs who came to India to bride-hunt, and would lament that they were forced to do so by the lack of eligible boys in town.[30]

Craig Jeffrey, in his ethnography *Timepass: Youth, Class and the Politics of Waiting in India*, observes a similar trend in North India:

Educated unemployed young men are often unable to marry. They frequently find it difficult to leave home and purchase or rent independent living space. [. . . And] are also commonly dogged by a sense of not having achieved locally salient norms of masculine success; they might conform by dint of their education to a particular vision of successful masculinity but lack the resources necessary to assume the role of male adult provider. Public discourses of educated unemployed young men as "louts" or hypermasculine and violent "threats" to the state and civil society exacerbate this gendered crisis.[31]

"Timepass" refers to the activities that the young men of Meerut would indulge in to kill time, which they had in plenty, given their unemployment. Jeffrey writes that "in contrast to the rich Jat farmers, who tended to imagine time as a commodity that should be 'invested,' many young men appeared to think of time as valueless—to be 'passed' or 'killed.'"[32]

I refer to these ethnographies on young men to convey the contradictions that they inhabit in rural India, where their lives unfold in gradual realizations that their time, space, and bodies are increasingly valueless; and further, to argue that hijras, in their hunger for cock and semen, provided a continued valorization of their semen and consolidated a masculinity that was fractured everywhere else. If fucking boys—*laudebaazi*—is the luxury (*shauk*) of the nawabs, then through fucking Azgari and other hijras, the boys enjoyed and tasted that luxury, wasting their precious semen that no one else in the world cared about past a certain point in time, not even their family, if it did not bring home the bread. In Ugra's homoerotic economy, the chocolate that is candy was offered to chocolates who are boys, in exchange for the pleasures of penetrating them. Chocolate as candy stands as a metonymy for childhood, a luxury for children; it was offered by Azgari's master and by the men in Ugra's short stories to boys, in exchange for fucking, which was a luxury, like chocolate, but for grown men. The failed subjectivity that defines hijras in their refusal to sublimate their sodomized histories and become the sodomizer—the fucker—and in remaining the fucked instead, offers the youths a chance to participate in another form of exchange. Azgari did not give chocolates to get "chocolates"; she would give chocolates and other little snacks to seduce young men—but then ask them to fuck her. In this economy she was giving chocolates and her "chocolate" to young men, who could not afford any form of luxury in the world. But what was she getting in return?

The protagonists in Ugra's short story "In Prison" have the following conversation:

"Once again, prisoners fought over a boy," replied the warder. "A Pathan threw down another Muslim man and bit off his nose with his teeth."

"For a boy!" I was surprised. "Are minors also kept in these prisons? Are there boys here too? Do noses get cut off and people get beaten over them here too?"

The warder replied, "Minors are not kept in this circuit, but who bothers about age in prison? Prisoners are long time sinners. Their boys can be anything up to sixty years old."[33]

Jaina was often called "grandmother" (*Jainani*) by people, and Azgari was often called "grandfather" (*Nana*), but never by the boys with whom they were having affairs, who were often decades younger than them. Jaina was seventy and Azgari sixty in 2013, and while they were treated with a lot of affection and respect by their lovers and other youths in Bhadrak, there was a noticeable lack of acknowledgment of their age in the everyday interactions between them. Azgari and Jaina never spoke about their age, or even referred to their aging bodies. I had been struck by the fact that the boys never made fun of them because of their age as they did with other old people roaming around the market. In the economy of giving chocolates and the pleasures of anal sex, hijras realigned their bodies as well as those of the youth to match the picture of pederasty. The boys became penetrating men with the luxury of dispensing semen and acquiring the truth about the world, and hijras remained young, like nubile "chocolates." Azgari's mythological frame of reference, then, highlighted the perpetual rottenness of the world that, though it had a larger claim on the oceanic water/semen of the boy, contradicted itself by no longer valuing it when it couldn't be transformed into other material values. Furthermore, the world reprimanded Azgari for spoiling the boy. What catastrophe would a small meal or a quiet fuck in the night in this cruel world have entailed? What did they get from creating a ruckus about the little pleasures of life?

The legacy of being penetrated is to teach how to become the penetrator, but in continuing to remain the penetrated, hijras' flesh—in Michael Moon's words—"stays weird." He writes:

Early in *In the Realms*, Darger writes that although some girls (and boys) may be weak and vulnerable, it is a widely known fact that the toughest girls are tougher than any boys. Who knows what early experiences of late fantasies of Darger's may subtend his confident assertion of this "fact"? Let us take the boy genitals with which he depicts so many of his "nuded" heroines as a sign that he declines to resolve the matter that vexes so many of his fellow pulp writers, the transformation of "weird flesh" . . . back into some normal state. Flesh in Darger tends to stay weird. Perhaps that is the most lasting sign of the legacy of pulp in his work—and of pulp's largely foreclosed promise of providing alternative histories of childhood and other conditions that Darger sees as forms of slavery, abuse, and atrocity.[34]

Hijras, whom I would like to see as heroines of Bhadrak, sometimes with boy's genitals, resemble Darger's "weird flesh" in many ways. Let me offer two ethnographic scenes to anchor my analogy.

I cannot remember when I got to know that the first person who fucked Bhatto was her maternal grandfather. Bhatto's mother had died, and she was sent to her maternal grandparents' place to live because her father had married again. I do remember asking Bhatto about it, and she would tell me amidst loud guffaws of laughter of how, when she was ten, her drunk grandfather had *done it* with her in the middle of the night. If we read this act of penetration in psychological terms, we could see Bhatto as struggling to return to a "normal state." Apart from the fact that Bhatto told me that because of her fucking grandfather she now preferred to have sex only with old men, I am hard-pressed to find evidence of a struggle, given that there was never any mention of moral outrage, let alone pain. It was an instance of flesh remaining weird, providing an alternative history to one of "abuse and atrocity." I am arguing that the failed pedagogy of penetration, that keeping on wanting to be fucked, keeps the flesh weird—and makes a hijra. Another instance of this keeping the flesh weird came from Akhtari, whom the other hijras used to mildly reproach for being in a relationship with her own nephew, her sister's son. When I asked what was wrong in getting fucked by your nephew, hijras who were gathered there discussing it told me, "He is a family man, and if his wife learns of it there will be a fight, she might leave him." When I asked who in the family could fuck them, the answer formed a pattern. It was not the male nephew from either side, either the husband of any female relative (sister, niece, mother, grandmother, daughter) or from men to whom they would have been nephews (FB, MB, MZH, FZH).[35] They could get fucked only by youths who were first cousins (FBS, MBS,

FZS, MZS)[36] and those cousin's sons—youths to whom they would be like grandparents (sons of their nieces and nephews from either side).

While sex between cousins was legitimized through cross-cousin marriage, the omission of a generation to allow sex only between one's grandfather's generation and one's grandson's generation—but not one's own grandfather or grandson obviously—is telling, not in its formulation but in its infringement. These rules were broken by Akhtari and by Bhatto, who was carrying on with her sister's husband. The reversal of the positions, to be fucked by the youth and not to fuck them, as Bhatto's grandfather did, I have argued, renders the sexual act a gesture of tenderness that consolidates the masculinity of the hungry, horny youth. But the breaking of the rules also gestured toward the rottenness of the laws of incest, the ones that are incipient to the social. Akhtari would often retort to the mild reproaches with smart, poetic comebacks like the following: "I tend to the tree, why should somebody else eat the fruit?" (*Gach hum lagaye, aur phal koi aur khayega?*), and "It's my possession, I know best how to take care of it" (*humara saaman hai, hum jaante hai kaise sambhalna*), and "why speak of nephews, I have no objections in getting fucked by my own son" (*bhanja, bhatija ka kya, mujhe apne ladke se bhi chudwane mein koi aitraaz nahin hai*). When one finds the whole world rotten, then why should one adhere to its rules? Invoking the rules of incest and then encouraging its transgression, but with the roles of penetration reversed, is the resistance that hijras offered through their failure, their subversive passivity, and their weird flesh. Akhtari and Bhatto show how laws of incest always have the subliminal possibility within them of being recognized precisely as a law in the act of transgression. This makes the rottenness of the world not an ontological given, but it is always available as a possible conclusion or as how it might as well have become completely rotten.

Let me clarify Moon's notion of weird flesh and its consonance with the love affairs between hijras and their lovers. In interpreting how Darger's heroines are endowed with what has been recognized as penises, Michael Moon repudiates psychologized readings, offering a more empirical analysis. He argues that given that Darger was tormented by the violence against little girls during his time, his drawing of ambiguous genitalia on the little girls in his artwork suggests that he imagined these girls to have the potential to refuse becoming victims in the way that being "little girls" implied, or in other words, to refuse being pathologized as little girls, and hence as victims. Comparing and contrasting Darger's superheroines with other superheroes of the time, Moon observes that while most superheroes transformed back into a normal state, the superheroines in Darger remained weird; that is, they never became little girls. This is the radical potential of Darger's paintings: the little girls didn't need to grow up or eventually become little girls; they could remain something else, something weird.[37] In Bhadrak, hijras like Bhatto, Akhtari, and Azgari refused as well to become victims of what could be easily read as pedophilia, incest, abuse, or trauma, and in fact by disavowing the language of pain, but by remaining penetrated, they became something other than a victim, something else, something weird—a hijra. What else would we call the form of carnality that does not register the breach of incest in expected ways? The weirdness is contagious, though, a contagion that I read as pedagogic because it imparts to the youth the lesson that the rules of the world are rules that can be broken. Let me offer some instances in which rules are meant to be broken in order to adhere to another set.

Varieties of incest, when committed, carried a variety of penalties in the various prescriptive texts of law, as would be expected. In tracing out this theme, I want to focus on a myth in the *Mahabharata* in which opprobrium is the consequence for not committing incest. The Indologist Wendy Doniger recounts the myth as follows:

> The celestial courtesan Urvasi fell in love with Arjuna and propositioned him, but he said she is like a mother to him and clapped his hands over his ears. Furious, the spurned nymph gave him a curse to be a dancer among women, devoid of honor, regarded as an impotent man (*kliba*). But Indra, the father of Arjuna, softened the curse and promised Arjuna that he would spend only a year as a dancer and then would be a man again. Years later, when it was time for Arjuna and his brothers to go into exile in disguise, Arjuna put on a woman's clothing (though he failed to disguise his hairy, brawny arms) and told his brothers: "I will be a *kliba*." He offered his services as a dancing master to the women in the harem of a king. The king was suspicious at first, remarking that Arjuna certainly did not look like a *kliba*, but he then ascertained that "her" lack of manhood was indeed firm and so let "her" teach his daughters to dance.[38]

Doniger compares this myth with others that are concerned with the transformation of women into men to point out a paradox: that is, "one Hindu view of gender makes it easy to slough off as pair of pants (or a dress), but this view is often challenged by myths in which skin is more than skin deep, in which the soul and the memory too are gendered, an intrinsic part of the moral coil that is not quite so easily shuffled off."[39]

But it is the psychoanalytical reading of this myth that makes it pertinent to hijras. Robert P. Goldman, in a magisterial essay, reads a large corpus of Hindu myths in the light of the Oedipal drama. The first intervention that he makes—and that I think should be pointed out here—is that of substitution. He writes, "It was in fact the recognition of such substitutions that led Freud to his most fundamental discoveries about the operation of the unconscious and therefore about the science of psychoanalysis itself. For it was his realization that the figures of friends, colleagues, etc., in his dreams and those of his patients were in fact representations of parental and other important figures that enabled him to produce *The Interpretation of Dreams*."[40] While acknowledging Goldman's groundbreaking analysis, James L. Fitzgerald substitutes *substitution* (pace Wittgenstein) for *resemblance* to offer a more anthropological reading of the Oedipal drama in the South Asian context. Fitzgerald argues that differentiating between *langue* and *parole* in the narratives of Indian families will enable us to see "elements that definitely resemble the classic 'Oedipal' triangle occur and recur in this story, but also . . . that these contribute only a part to some larger tableau of meaning that can be ethically construed in pragmatic social settings."[41]

Here I rely on Fitzgerald's argument to make my point that it is not important that hijras followed a certain generational distance to calibrate the incest taboo. This is not only because hijras in their families substituted for and resembled figures of authority—especially to their grandnephews—but because they broke the taboo all the time and faced only mild reproach. If they broke one formulation of the incest taboo to adhere to another, then we could have argued that they were legitimizing some form of intimacy to serve a larger purpose: Hindu rules of leviratic marriages and other *niyojana* rules of procreation are examples of this. But because they were breaking all the rules of incest, including the ones that they themselves had set up, they were signaling a different realization of the world—a realization that all rules can be broken and that all rules rot the flesh.

Let us go back to the myth of Arjuna's refusal to commit incest to clarify what I mean. Goldman has read that particular myth to consolidate his argument concerning the existence of the Oedipal drama in Indian narratives. He sees Arjuna's refusal to have sex with his ancestress as the renunciation of the mother who is the sexual object of the Oedipal rivalry, thereby resulting in a negative Oedipal resolution, which is the passive homosexual identification with the father.[42] Fair enough, but if Bersani insists that there is resistance in this failure—and I have argued that this resistance is pedagogical—then what can the incest enacted by Akhtari and Bhatto, reversing the roles in incestuous fucking, teach? What does it mean to be fucked by your grandson rather than fucking him? Why is Arjuna cursed for refusing to commit incest?

The reason for this is to be found in another set of texts according to which these men have broken one set of rules in view of upholding another. Siegel, in his study of the *Gita Govinda*, cites Sir John Woodroffe's *Introduction to Tantra Sastra*: "It is said in *Sruti*, '*talpagatam na pariharet*' (she who comes to your bed is not to be refused), for the rule of chastity that is binding him [the *yogin*] yields to such an advance on the part of a woman."[43] This rule, according to tantric texts, extends to one's mother and sister and is a component of profaning rituals that are sacred or part of sacred rituals that are profane. Although Siegel employs the words *sacred* and *profane*, scholars after Siegel have argued that this dichotomy hardly works in the South Asian context.[44] To cite Siegel again:

> A passage in the *Tantras* instructs the initiate to indulge in forbidden, sexual, incestuous, blasphemous activity in order to secure liberation: "inserting his organ into the mother's womb, pressing his sister's breasts, placing his foot upon his *guru's* head, he will be reborn no more." Perhaps this means simply that he who is liberated is beyond all morality, all good and evil, beyond even *dharma*; but the verse is also taken by commentators to be written in a code language, the "twilight language" or "intentional language," *sandhya-bhasa*.[45]

Siegel goes on to offer an analysis that reads the tantric passage cited allegorically, building on previous scholarship that has seen it as a coded reference to yogic practices, where the mother's womb refers to "*muladhara* or base centre of the yoga body, the sister's breasts are the heart and the throat centre (*anahata* and *ajna*) respectively, and the guru's head is the brain centre"[46]—thus translating it as instructions for a yogi. Without discounting this reading, I want to ask what the use of such metaphors implies and if we can actually read incest performed by hijras as a way of teaching

her nephews and grandsons to be beyond dharma, liberated from and beyond morality. While I am questioning the reliance on merely metaphoric
incest in tantric sex, David Gordon White, in studying a subgenre of tantric sex, the *kaula*, questions whether it is only a metaphoric reliance. He
writes, "The tendency toward a literalization of symbolic statements or practices is one that David Shulman has also identified as a hallmark of many
extreme forms of south Indian devotionalism. Most importantly, . . . much
of the Tantric terminology makes sense only if it is read literally; indeed, I
would argue that the ritual edifice of early Tantra only stands, that early Tantra only functions as a coherent system, if these terms are put into literal
practice."[47] Though hijras are not tantrics, can we see in the incest performed
by hijras—in which they seduce youths to whom they are related and are
penetrated by them—as a pedagogy of a different sort: not of yogic emancipation but of teaching the ways of the world in which consolidating masculinity needs to go beyond strict laws of dharma and morality. If such
instructions can only utilize metaphors of incest, then actual incest must
be imagined as a practice of some value other than that of immorality. This
brings us back to the economy of semen and the way value is imparted to it
in the practice of ritualized tantric sex, either through allegorical or actualized incest.

I offer a very truncated version of tantric sex as studied and summarized
by David Gordon White in his masterful study *Kiss of the Yogini*. This summary will also explicate the tantric philosophy only hinted at by Siegel. Very
briefly, yoginis are a set of semidivine goddesses, an externalized form of the
godhead, who are embodied in human women and who, through being possessed by the goddesses, according to White, "carried in their bodies the
germ plasm of the godhead, called the 'clan fluid' (*kuladravyam*), 'clan nectar' (*kulamrta*), 'vulval essence' (*yonitattva*), or simply the 'fluid' (*dravyam*),
or the 'clan' (*kula*)." While this fluid essence of the godhead flowed naturally
through these female beings, it was absent in males.[48] The "son of the clan" or
kulaputra is required to have sex with yoginis, offering them his semen in
exchange for the germ plasm that flows through the sexual fluids, or lotus
juice, of the women. These yoginis are also related to the mother goddesses
and can be seen as ancestresses of clans who must be pleased through the
offering of semen. While the women of the clan are obviously the bearers of
children, they are not seen to carry the clan fluid; it can only be passed
through the men, who acquire it through having sex with yoginis. These

goddesses, if not pleased, will devour the infants of the clan and must be pacified for the safe birth and life of the clan's children. Related to ensuring the safety of the progeny of men, the yoginis impart to the men supernatural powers, which explains the patronage offered to tantra by kings looking to consolidate and amplify the power of kingship. White writes that "later Tantric sexual practice came to be grounded in a theory of transformative aesthetics, in which the experience of orgasm effected a breakthrough from 'contracted' self-consciousness to an expansive 'god consciousness,' in which the entire universe came to be experienced as 'self.'"[49]

Hijras, like yoginis, by seducing men and breaking the rules of incest, by "feeding" on their semen, would in the view of the people in Odisha give the men supernatural powers. Very much like Darger's heroines, yoginis and hijras keep the flesh weird and, by making the flesh of their men weird, make them into superhuman men and ward off their being cursed with impotence. Serena Nanda offers an ethnographic example that can tie all of this together.

> Sushila spoke very warmly of her husband and was disconsolate because she could not give him a child. She very much wanted this for him, because she thought it was necessary that he lead "a normal family life." . . . When I returned to Bastipore in the summer of 1985, Sushila had quite an achievement to tell me about. She was now a mother-in-law and a grandmother! How had this come about? "She proudly told me that she had adopted her [former] husband as her son and had arranged his marriage with a neighbour's sister. The girl was poor, but respectable, and quite pretty. The couple now had a son, making Sushila a grandmother. They were living with the boy's mother in another part of the city, but they visited Sushila nearly every day and I often met with them. Since her "son's" marriage Sushila had found another husband, a man who does not live with her but often comes to spend the night.[50]

Nanda's informant Sushila transformed her sexual affair with her husband into incest but did so out of a desire to give the man a child, a family, and thus consolidate his *kula*. This was something that would surely require superhuman powers in face of all the adversities—such as the curses of impotence and child mortality because of devouring mother goddesses—that can befall a man trying to create a family and continue his lineage, institutions that are as suffocating in their fragility as in their ideology.

Another set of narratives of love affairs between hijras and their men shows the damages that follow from transforming lovers into sons. Hijras, even if they are similar to yoginis in their power to transform men into superhumans through transactions in semen, and also similar to Darger's heroines in keeping their flesh weird and making the flesh of their lovers weird as well, are after all human. In the following ethnographic narratives, I attempt to show the aftermath of love affairs. Masterani, a hijra in Jajpur, would spend the entire night on the phone with her lover. All the hijras of Jajpur used to sleep in one room in their hijra guru's house. Guruma used to sleep in another room, and Radha got a separate room because she was the senior-most *cela*. While I was living there I was given a blanket and asked to sleep in the communal room, as well. Masterani would cover her head with the blanket, and we would overhear soft mutterings, cooings, and murmurings from underneath the blanket throughout the night. After a few days I caught her alone and asked her about the one who had stolen the sleep of her nights. Masterani blushed and said, "I had gone to Talcher to visit a friend and I saw this young man there. I asked my friend to get his number because I fell in love with him as soon as I saw him. I called him and soon we were talking all the time and we fell in love. When I was twelve years old I decided that I wanted to marry a man who must realize how much love I have for him in my heart. I don't care if he keeps a physical relation, but he must recognize what's in my heart. You won't believe how much I love him. If a child shits on his mother's lap, will the mother cut away her limb? No, she won't mind it at all; she will calmly clean it and then take the child back onto her lap. Just like that I love him; even if he shits on me, I will like it. I will never get angry but will continue to love him."

The analogy struck me as odd, and the more I thought about it, the more I realized why it had seemed to me a bit misplaced. Usually a mother's love is viewed in contradistinction to the erotic love of a wife—blood versus sexuality—but in Masterani's usage this distinction was collapsed; the singularity of a mother's love for her child was used as an analogy and measure by which to compare the erotic love that she felt for this man. The degree of her love was not made comprehensible in terms of gods and devotees (analogies used by Nanda's hijra), or master and servant, or husband and wife—but mother and child. In fact, Masterani used to say, "I want to be his brother, sister, mother, father, friend, everything." She would often use the example of a child shitting on a parent's lap to explain the inevitable betrayals, disappointments, and pitfalls that accompany all types of intimacy in and with this world. For example, she would say that a hijra could never love another hijra completely: "If you shit on your mother's lap will she cut the limb away; no, she will continue to love you; but hijras, if you so much as fart in their presence, will kick you out of the house."

I begin my analysis with this story of being everything to the lover to show the damages that accrue from being everything to someone—mother and wife, brother and sister, father and friend—and of not getting angry at your lover for shitting on you. A myth that was told to me gives form to this impossible task of being everything to one's lover and of obliterating the self's boundaries in love. In order to relate that myth that was told to me in connection with hijras' desire for a lover—"husband fever"[51]—I must first recount the myths of Bahuchara Mata, the patron goddess of hijras, which have been recorded by scholars and were told to me as well. The first myth is as follows:

Bahuchara was a pretty, young maiden in a party of travelers passing through the forest in Gujarat. The party was attacked by thieves, and fearing that they would outrage her modesty, Bahuchara drew her dagger and cut off her breast, offering it to the outlaws in place of her virtue. This act, and her ensuing death, led to Bahuchara's deification and the practice of self-mutilation and sexual abstinence by her devotees to secure her favor. Bahuchara is also specifically worshipped by childless women in the hope of bearing a child, particularly a son.[52]

The second myth is as follows:

In one story, a king prayed to Bahuchara for a son. She granted him his wish, but his son, named Jetho, was impotent. One night Bahuchara appeared in a dream and commanded Jetho to cut off his genitals, dress in female clothing, and become her servant. Jetho obeyed the goddess and from that time on, it is said, impotent men get a call from the goddess in their dreams to be emasculated. Indeed, there is a belief in Gujarat that impotent men who resist the call of Bahuchara to get emasculated will be born impotent for seven future births.[53]

The third myth, recorded in slightly different versions by Reddy and Nanda, is as follows:

> Once there was a prince whose parents wanted to get him married. The boy did not want to get married, but his parents insisted. They selected this goddess as his wife, and the marriage took place. He was a very handsome boy, but the Mata was also a very beautiful lady. But after the marriage the husband and wife never joined together. On the first night, leaving the goddess alone in the nuptial room, the prince rode away into the forest. The goddess waited till dawn and felt very angry that her husband had left her. This went on for some months. The goddess felt very hurt and decided to investigate. So one night she followed him on a path to the forest clearing where the prince had been acting like the hijras. She was puzzled by what she had seen and returned home. When her husband returned, she said to him, "I want to ask you something, do not get angry at me. Don't you feel that you must have your wife by you?" Then the prince fell at her feet and told her, "Mother, if I had the urge for a wife and children I wouldn't have left you and gone away. I am neither a man nor a woman, and that is the truth." The goddess got very angry and said, "They have spoiled my life by hiding the facts, and therefore your life will also be spoiled. Hereafter, people like you should be *nirvan* [undergo emasculation in order to be reborn]." So saying, she cut off his genitals. After cutting off his genitals she said, "people like you, who are going to have this *nirvan*, should call me at that time." After this the prince took on the form of a woman.[54]

Invoking these myths will help make sense of the myth that was told to me by Madhubai when she was trying to explain why hijras' relationships with their men failed and inevitably ended. She said:

> Bahuchara Mata is neither man nor woman. She didn't have any family; she had not married, and didn't have children. She had no desire for anybody, she was *nishkama* (without desire) and would roam around singing *kirtans* and begging; whatever she would earn from begging, she would cook and eat at night. Once she was roaming around begging from house to house, singing and clapping her hands. A hijra child who had been born in a house in that village heard Mata clapping and came

running to her and told her, "I want to be like you, take me around with you." So Bahuchara Mata took her and they started living together. Once this cela was roaming around with Mata, she fell in love with a boy, a son of a Rajput family. Knowing that love and desire was forbidden to her, the cela transformed her lover into a mosquito and hid him in her coiffure. Later that night when Bahuchara Mata and her cela returned home, Mata put out two plates for dinner and two plates ended up becoming three. Every time she would put out two plates, it would become three. She asked her cela why this was happening? The cela said she didn't know and couldn't tell. The Mata got angry and grabbed the cela's hair; the coiffure came undone and the mosquito flew out. She understood immediately that the cela had fallen in love and recognized the mosquito as the Rajput boy. She told her cela, "What you have done is not right, you have given your mind and body to somebody else. I cannot live here, I am going to Patal,"[55] and she cursed the cela by saying: "In Kaliyuga, you hijras will find it as difficult to find a lover as it is to catch a mosquito. The cela cried out, "Mata, how can you leave me like this, how will I live? How will I eat? You cannot leave like this." As the Mata was going down to Patal, the cela grabbed her hair and Mata said, "Just as you heard my claps and came to me, so will others come hearing your clap, and that's how you will also find celas. You will be castrated, you will not live happily with your lingas, and you will earn your life through begging. You will keep your hair long like mine so that people may pull your hair as you are pulling mine."

I want to read the narratives of love stories that were told to me, as well as the narratives recorded by Nanda and Reddy in their ethnographies, in light of this myth—that is, that finding and keeping a lover is like trying to catch hold of a mosquito, nearly impossible. Reddy is puzzled by the resilience of hijras' desire for a husband/lover in the face of glaring evidence that shows it is impossible. She writes, "Given the ubiquity of abuse, violence, and abandonment, as well as hijra/kotis' ambivalence toward men in general, why this strong desire for a social *jodi* (bond)? Why do kotis have such an overwhelming need for a loving husband?"[56] She tracks through an exhaustive array of literature, and I quote at length the conclusion she reaches to explain the yearning for a husband and lover, when one knows that the search will almost inevitably end in betrayal and failure.

If desire or love plays a central role in the lives of hijras and kotis, it is through the various, ambiguous, and conflicting patterns of kinship . . . that this love is made manifest. Only through understanding the relations between the idealized systems of kinship that hijras and kotis hold to, and the nature of desire and lived experience in which these ideals are often not sustained, can we *begin* to comprehend the "local pleasures and afflictions" and the cultural patternings of their lives.[57]

Let me offer, then, some scenes that will clarify the pattern according to which love affairs unfolded amongst hijras in Bhadrak and Bhawanipatna. This pattern does not deviate from the ones recorded so faithfully by Nanda and Reddy. One evening, Nandita and I were cycling around in Bhawanipatna when she said, "Listen, my husband has asked me for 25,000 rupees; do you think I should give it to him?" She asked the question in a tone of indecision, and I used it to air what I had been wondering about concerning material transactions in love affairs, which was a constant trope when these affairs were recounted, usually in terms of use, abuse, and exploitation. I asked, "Why don't you want to give it? If you love him and he loves you, who else will he turn to if he needs the money; he can't ask strangers for help, he will obviously ask you, and if you love him, who else will you give the money to?" Nandita remained silent and said, "You are right, he is my husband, if he doesn't ask me who else will he ask?" Damru's friends would also constantly warn her that Damru shouldn't spend so much money on her lover, whom she was trying very hard to seduce—he hadn't slept with her as yet. Friends would tell her that men would just use her for money and would leave her when she wouldn't be able to give them anything. Damru blew up one day; since I was the one with her, she turned to me and screamed, "Why shouldn't I give him anything? Everybody gives their boyfriends all sorts of things—they buy them motorcycles, clothes, everything—why shouldn't I also give my boyfriend things?"

There was a pattern to which all love stories conformed in Bhawanipatna and Bhadrak. Hijras would often seduce men by giving them presents. These presents would create the largest dent in their budgets; they would work very hard—or steal, borrow, or beg from friends—to buy their lovers presents that would range from everyday things like clothes, food, and beer to more expensive things such as watches, motorcycles, tuition for computer classes, and so on. Reddy offers ethnographic narratives of kotis who had even sold their kidneys for their lovers. "Frank, a middle-aged, Christian man in his mid-forties, had suffered untold hardships for his pantis. He had sold his blood to a blood bank, and later his kidney, to earn enough money to satisfy his current panti. He had lost several jobs on account of 'his man,' been physically abused, and suffered ill health after the sale of his kidney."[58] The mortification of Frank's flesh can be seen as nothing but the carnality of kinship; but the difference between kinship and love in this instance lay in the fact that the bodies of hijras, after their monetary value had been squeezed out, were depleted of value—forgotten and abandoned—whereas in kinship the bodies became old, animal-like, part of lineage, and if they were forgotten and abandoned, it was accompanied with opprobrium. There was no invocation of a morality breach here, explained by "Alzheimers, the bad family, and other modern things"; instead, there was puzzlement. Damru once asked me, "Why do they do this to us, don't their hearts pain them when they do this?" I turned and looked ahead because I didn't have an answer, and Damru said, "Well, this is what lovers do."

If guilt and shame can be attached to kin for their betrayal and ill-treatment of their family members, their absence here forces us to reevaluate the pattern of love affairs: What exactly accounts for the impossibility of finding a lover to whom you are everything, of catching a mosquito? Hijras would begin their love affairs by spending all their hard-earned money on their lovers. One night a hijra whispered to me about another, "She has even bought a car for her husband." The extent to which they converted their entire existence into money and other gifts for their lovers was often recounted to me either by them, when remarking on their lover's betrayal, or by their friends in melancholic awe. Damru told me that Pawan hijra, who had a hard time earning money in the first place, given that she was not the most sought-after hijra prostitute, had "pawned her cell phone, sold off her cooking stove and cycle and other things that she possessed so that she could have some money to give to her then lover, Sonu." Pawan hijra would rob from her clients; if they took her to their houses she would steal anything and everything she could lay her hands on so that she could sell them and give the money to her lover. She would often be caught and beaten up; given that she stole property from her own home—such as the gas cylinder, stove, jewelry, and so on—her brothers would also beat her up upon discovery. In Reddy's ethnography, the property that was placed for sale extended to hijras' and kothis' blood and kidneys, as well.

While hijras were warned and reproached for putting everything up for sale, they were also discredited if they did not go beyond themselves for their lovers. After fucking Nandita, Sajjan confessed that he had borrowed 30,000 from his father and spent it, so he doesn't know what to do. I said to Nandita, "He didn't ask you for money, so why are you upset?" Nandita replied, "But he said it in a way so as to imply that he wanted me to give it to him." Nandita took this disillusionment with Sajjan very badly and vowed never to take his calls and to forget him; she abused him for being selfish. Damru made quite a lot of fun of her behind her back: "Look she kept on chanting his name, 'Sajjan, Sajjan . . .' but in the end he wants her money, and she can't even give it to him—she wanted to make him her husband and she couldn't even give her husband 30,000—what sort of love is this?" I found it interesting that Damru both criticized Sajjan for asking for money, thus casting a doubt over his love for Nandita, and criticized Nandita for refusing to give it: "You can't even give money to the man you love; the man you want to make your husband."

There would be a point beyond which hijras would not be able to sell anything, but the lovers who were now seduced by gifts would keep on demanding money and presents. The love affair would start with hijras surprising the men with a gift, the number of gifts would increase, the love affair would be consummated when an especially large request of the lover was fulfilled; for a while gifts were given and requests met, but when the requests kept on coming and hijras were no longer able to satisfy them, a point was reached where the lover had to prove that his love was true and not just pure greed. At this point hijras would not give anything more, would withdraw all their material support, and would expect the lovers to remain with them in spite of not getting any material benefits. This was the moment that Nandita had reached with her husband, who had asked her for 25,000 rupees; she was wondering whether he was with her because she gave him money or because he truly loved her. As Michael Hardt writes:

The expression "for love or money" is generally used to indicate the two extremes, which cover between them the entire spectrum. "I wouldn't do that for love or money" means I wouldn't do that in exchange for anything. It can be interesting, however, to read that *or* as marking not an opposition but a common function that love and money share, somewhat like the *or* in Spinoza's famous phrase "deus sive natura" which claims polemically, that god and nature are two names for substance itself. I do not intend to propose that love and money are the same thing, but rather, that putting them in relation can reveal the power to create and maintain social bonds that is proper to money and can (and perhaps should) be also the vocation of love. Posing love in relation to the power of money can help us construct a properly political concept of love.[59]

I will argue shortly that the love affairs conducted in the form that they are by hijras are the exercise—though often met with failure—of a concept of love that can have certain political implications. Before I do that, I want to place the love affairs in Bhadrak and Bhawanipatna alongside Hardt's line of argument, which does not view love and money as an opposition but as sharing a common function of valuation. Lauren Berlant, in her commentary on Michael Hardt's argument, writes, "What could interrupt the translation of all social relations into propertied ones? What other kinds of infrastructure for proximity can develop that will bind us to the world in which we find each other; or bind us to each other and, in such binding, make a world? It's hard even to lasso the right phrases together to get the rhythms of sociality in sufficient sync to render a habitable material present, or world."[60] The transactional logic of the love affairs conducted by hijras is inverse to the logic commented on by Hardt and Berlant, hence its political ramifications are both apparent and not. The love affairs did not attempt to translate social relations into propertied ones but to translate the exchange of properties such as kidneys, blood, and other gifts into a social relation that belonged to another world. The gifts and presents were not exchanges calibrated according to the logic of kin-making but were more similar to—though slightly different from—the logic of potlatch. Hijras would go beyond what they could afford and what was considered appropriate to collect money and buy presents for their lovers. They would sell their bodies, kidneys, blood; they would beg, borrow, and steal to buy quotidian objects that their lovers, who were young men, desired: cars, motorbikes, cellphones, clothes, objects that were circulated in advertisements and markets and worked as markers of masculinity, class, respect, and power.

The hardships hijras faced in procuring the requisite amount of money was often recounted in stories of a battle proudly fought. After a point, the lovers were expected to respond, to reciprocate, not similarly in kind, as in a potlatch, but similarly in spirit. They were to give love that was equivalent to the love of hijras, not by giving presents but by loving that went beyond any material profit. They were required to mortify their flesh and souls by giving love that had no anchor in the material world—a love without benefits, a love without price. Equivalent, because if a hijra's mode caused her body to disintegrate by placing itself completely in the market, where everything is bought and sold, then the lover was expected to disintegrate his body by refusing any comfort that comes with translating that love into property, or worse, profit. This was seen in Masterani's demand that she be everything to her lover—mother, father, brother, sister, and friend. If one acquiesces to have just one social relation and then refuses to translate that into a propertied one, the transformation of the self required is nothing if not tremendous, and as Berlant writes, "In the vernacular of love it is impossible to tell the difference between destructive and world-building impulses. We see that revolutionary impulses are destructive, too, but the spin it puts on that points to productive destruction (of the mommy-daddy-me machine, and yet families are still the fundamental imaginary and economic unit)."[61]

Mangu introduced me to Biju and her husband, Dhabala, in the summer of 2009. Mangu probably took me there because I would constantly ask questions about love, and given that she did not have a husband or paramour, she was quite indifferent and unsympathetic to my cynicism and desperation for love. She took me to Biju's hut, and I started asking them about their relationship. Ten years ago, Biju and several other hijras had gone to Dhabala's village to dance at a religious festival to earn some money. Dhabala fell in love with her, and they got married the next morning at a nearby temple; he left his family and home to be with her. Dhabala's parents and brothers didn't stop him; they had two other sons, and he had seen them only once, three years ago, since he got married. Dhabala accompanies Biju when she goes to dance and play the *dholak* at weddings, religious festivals, and childbirths. This relation would have approximated the idea of world-making that Masterani and other hijras wanted, in which one social relation suffuses the whole world and is valuable beyond price. In the years since, Biju started drinking hooch very heavily, and in 2013, when I finally caught up with her, she was drunk at eight o'clock in the morning. I had heard about her drinking and the consequent fighting with Dhabala over the years. Varsha told me that last year Biju had fallen unconscious once near the railway tracks foaming at the mouth because of adulterated hooch. Dhabala had taken her to the hospital and taken care of her. I asked Varsha why Biju drank so much. Varsha said, "Biju needs to be drunk to go begging on the trains; her husband told her that she doesn't need to beg if she has to drink to be able to do it. He started earning income by selling boiled eggs at the train station, but after three or four months Biju started drinking again." Varsha did not have any answers as to why Biju drank so much when her husband told her that she doesn't need to beg.

I grabbed Biju's hand and asked, "What's going on? Everybody has told me that you are drinking so much. Dhabala loves you so much, why are you trying to ruin such a beautiful love? Will you like it if he leaves you?" Biju's skin had discolored, and she had become bloated and looked very unhappy. She just smiled, kissed me on my cheek, and got on the train. I offer this ethnographic narrative to underscore Berlant's ambivalence about love that is not dependent on being translated into property. It might be seen as destructive, or more accurately, a failed attempt at remaking a world. Hardt writes, "Love is thus always a risk in which we abandon some of our attachments to this world in the hope of creating another, better one." Hardt's essay argues for transformative love from a reading of Marx; it can be argued that Biju and Dhabala lost that wager in a way, but in comparison to other failures hijras met with in their quest to catch mosquitoes—to forge a social relation that would resist any kind of propertied or even material translation—Biju and Dhabala would still count as a success, but perhaps not of the kind we expected. Berlant warns us about this expectation, "if we could cluster around it [love] a genuinely realistic and visionary set of transformations that do not overstate the consoling promises that sacrifice the human to an idealized vision."[62] If our expectations are just that the lovers of hijras do not consider hijra bodies expendable and dispensable— painful stories of which abound—then love did not transform Biju and Dhabala's world to the extent that money was replaced by love. Hardt writes further:

> Love or money, Marx tells us, that is our choice. It is significant in my view that, by establishing this alternative, Marx poses love on the same level of money: love operates not only in terms of intimate relations but also in a primary role of social organization. This same comparison, however, diminishes the power of love, in my view, insofar as it leads Marx to consider love only in terms of exchange. "If you love unrequitedly,"

he writes, "i.e. if your love as love does not call forth love in return, if through the *vital expression* of yourself as a loving person you fail to become a *loved person*, then your love is impotent, it is a misfortune."[63]

Besides Biju and Dhabala's love affair, most other affairs were impotent; they did not result in the loving person becoming a loved person. Nanda wrote of one such affair. "Even though she had an educated husband, he would eat off her hands only and didn't contribute toward the household expenses. This made Kamladevi fall ill, and she had had asthma before, so she passed away."[64] I was frequently told about Suman, whom I had met in 2009 but who died in 2011, before I returned to Bhawanipatna. When I returned and inquired about Suman, a vivacious personality—funny, beautiful, and charming—and we had become very fond of each other, I was told that she had sold everything off for her lover, her little eatery, her jewelry, and when she lay dying her husband abandoned her and went back to his parents. Hijras were acutely aware of the impotence of lovers; when a man didn't get what he wanted from one hijra, he would try his luck with others.

Rajeshwari had a boyfriend, Bulu, but she realized that he was only after her money. Sapna seduced him by giving him what he wanted. He then demanded 7,000 rupees for a mobile phone, but after promising him the money, Sapna found herself unable to give it to him. Now Bulu is calling one hijra after another in Bhawanipatna, offering his services and beauty in order to find a more generous patron. Each hijra whom he called made false promises that she would give him the money and have sex with him. They laugh behind his back and say, "We told him yes, we will give you the money, let us suck your cock, and then we just don't receive his calls." The lover who does not rise to the challenge of reciprocating the generosity of spirit of hijras with a generosity of his own—a generosity that resists the translation of social relations into material ones—becomes as impotent as a hijra: used, abused, and a joke.

Michael Hardt, analyzing Marx's brief comments on love, writes:

Love, like the other senses, is conceived as a social organ, or really a human power to create social bonds. Like new powers to see and think we also must gain a new power to love. Perhaps we should call these social "muscles," rather than "organs," because we develop them through use and practice, breaking them down and building them up to strengthen and expand our human relations to the world, that is, our powers to create and manage social bonds. The development of a new sensorium, increasing our power to love and the strength of the other social muscles, is inversely related to the rule of private property.[65]

Hardt's reading of love is strikingly congruent with the spiritual exercises of Sufism, which were taught through tales of Hindavi romances. These two disparate literary sources have in common the faith that love transforms; they also both contend that the new form taken by the transformation of the self and the world is not known; its potentiality is signaled, and its need is felt—but is it inevitably marked with failure, as an impossible place to go, or rather an impossible task to achieve—like catching a mosquito? Lawrence Cohen remarks on Michael Hardt's delicious proposition and brings it closer to the geometry of love that I am drawing. He writes, "The only love worth its name is not that which can be bought but that which has been achieved through a worked-on self encountering its equal in labor."[66]

I will defend my use of the word *geometry* when I draw a parallel between the spiritual exercises of Sufism as allegorized through romantic love and the exercises of valuation, labor, and exchange as undertaken by hijras. Cohen has already initiated this parallelism by using the phrase "not that which can be bought." This is precisely what hijras desired, a love from their lovers that cannot be bought through gifts or the exchange of presents but one that necessarily passes through those points to reveal the extent to which hijras' body, labor, time, and effort were at the disposal of their lovers. These notions of stages, or points of revelation and recognition, are also words that code the ostensibly ornate romances as pedagogic tools of Sufi spiritualism. Cohen raises the possibility of such a love affair. Is it possible to catch a mosquito? Is it possible for anybody, let alone the lovers of hijras, to respond in a way that goes beyond the triad "of family, property, and honor"? He observes, "If, for a time, homosex was good to think as a figure exercising a conception of love beyond property and the nation, it was as most figures are for some people and not others and with a series of gendered effects. Its ability to stand for an alternate present, let alone another future, was limited. But perhaps we ask too much of organs like love, even that nonunified true love we do not yet know, to give us the positive transformation to come."[67]

Love and its promise of a transformed world that is palpable and can be achieved through the exercise of spiritual muscles were the foundation of the Sufi romances of sultanate India. Aditya Behl, in his posthumous publication *Love's Subtle Magic: An Indian Islamic Literary Tradition, 1379–1545*, writes, "The poets of the Hindavi Sufi romances commonly use the phrase 'the shadow of paradise on earth' (*janu kabilasa utari bhui chava*) to describe elements of their fictional landscapes. . . . These references to shadows of an elusive paradise are the hallmark of a genre of Sufi romance that is assumed to put forward 'the equation of human love and love for a divine being.'"[68] Hijras, in asking of their lovers a love that resists transformation into materiality/property, were in effect asking for a paradise whose shadows can be felt on earth. It is the same paradise the possibility of which Hardt is arguing, one in which lovers are asked to have a stake in each other at a register that overrides exchange, circulation, and economy, or in Simmel's terms, that resists the slide from value to price. The manner in which hijras staked their bodies for their lovers could be seen also as an emotional-spiritual exercise, analogous to the ones that the heroes of Sufi romances undertake. The romances, though, always end happily in various forms of mystical annihilation, *fanaa*, when the lovers have achieved a certain spiritual enlightenment after having purged themselves of the baser elements of human desire, thereby distilling themselves into appropriate mirrors of godhood and love. *Fanaa*, at least in one form, does not allow itself to be translated as an experience of radical alterity resulting from an asceticism that takes one out of this world. When he juxtaposes the many Sufi romances vis-à-vis each other, Behl highlights that *fanaa* is accessible to all and does not require one to sacrifice one's world, but rather to transcend it: "The only annihilation is of the seeker's own carnal nature, which gives him the concrete power simultaneously to stay in the world and to transcend it."[69] Hijras, in asking their lovers to purge themselves of their carnal nature, signal toward the shadows of paradise, which can transform this world into something else—an impossibility, perhaps, but a task worth undertaking.

Mohammad Habib, in his essay "Early Muslim Mysticism," offers a translation of *fanaa* that not only reveals the manner in which it was grafted on to the South Asian context but renders it less esoteric than it reads in Behl's work. He writes, "To the *Kharrazis* or followers of Abu Sa'id Kharraz belongs the credit of having restated the age-old conception of *nirvana*, the expansion (not annihilation, as is sometimes supposed) of the human soul into the Absolute."[70] Thus *fanaa*, or the spiritual exercises of the Sufis, referred to annihilation not in any dramatic way but rather in the gradual manner that the soul expands limitlessly by being attached to the Absolute.

Fanaa does mean annihilation, but only in the sense that the soul does not remain as it was previously—in other words, it becomes weird. Through their relentless fucking, hijras, with their contagious weird flesh, would in a way reveal to the youth that the rules of this world do not exhaust it. That there is a margin between the rules and the world and that another form of being can be achieved is possible by recognizing that gap.

I have used the word *geometry* here to signal a similarity between the patterns of Sufi romances and the love affairs of hijras: the birth of desire, the claims of love, the mortification of flesh in the service of this love, the disappointing failures or the misfortunes of love, which refer to men not recognizing the potential of love to transcend this world—or, in Hardt's words, to transform the world. In his essay "The Symmetry of *Madhumalati*" (appended to Behl's translation of the text), Simon Weightman organizes the narrative into points of coincidence and opposition to write, "The story is circular and a brief scrutiny of other Shattari works reveals that the circle was their favourite and most persistent symbol used in expressing the cosmology of the Order as well as in many other applications."[71] The following (Figure 1) is a graphic representation of the symmetry as drawn by Weightman. Through delineating several geometric patterns embedded in them, Weightman has forcefully argued its consonance with tantric symbolism. Both Behl and Weightman have studied Sufi romances to argue for a certain mutual intelligibility achieved during the Delhi sultanate era, between Hindu and Islamic philosophies, through the creation of texts such as *Madhumalati*. I cite their work in order to recognize love affairs between hijras and their men/husbands/lovers as an exercise similar to spiritual ones that probe the possibility of transcending or transforming the experience of this world.

This transcendence and transformation are also a part of the romance, as Weightman has noted, though in this religious work it is more concerned with God than with men. Reddy's informant, Frank, in giving a narrative of his love affair, says, "'I adored you, I worshipped you,' I said, 'You are my god. My people know, but my people are not proud of you. . . . Okay, I walked out of my house because of you. I left my house because of you. I left my family because of you. I left my friends because of you, I left my neighbours because of you, I left my cousins, my aunties, my uncles, *everybody* I left because of you. I'm living *alone* because of you.'"[72] Nanda's informant tells her, "But Ahmed is like a God to me, because when he came back he saved me from all this humiliation. . . . God and he are one to me. I used to be so thin, as thin as Sushila. I had asthma, and I was always short of breath. Ahmed didn't mind that at all but would always make me sleep beside him."[73] Pawan hijra once got frustrated with my constant probing regarding the way hijras would put everything in the service of their lovers and said, "When a hijra falls in love, her *panthi* becomes her god. She doesn't look left, she doesn't look right; if her man says, it is morning when it is night, she will believe it is morning. She goes mad."

The Sufi romances are an allegory of the relationship between a novice and his God; he has to love God, who in the narrative is revealed as a woman with divine beauty, and uniting with her would result in the experience of *fanaa*—a world that transcends the current base one. The love affairs in rural Odisha were mimetic of this allegory: lovers became gods, but unfortunately there were a lot of false gods out there. Weightman takes the pattern cited and highlights yet another pattern in it: the yogic symbol of the *coincidentia oppositorum* of love, and now the Shattari Sufi cosmology. Paul Kockelman's essay "Value Is Life under an Interpretation: Existential Commitments, Instrumental Reasons and Disorienting Metaphors" allows me to expand the similarities I have drawn between the Sufi/yogic exercises and the love affairs of hijras. Until now I have argued that both forms of spiritual exercises imagined that a different regime of valuation was achievable; this was also the potential of love held out by Hardt and the hope or the good faith with which hijras fell in love. Kockelman's essay uses maps as the metaphor to shed light on how value is imparted, arranged, and most importantly interpreted. He writes, "One weighs the relative desirability of possible paths by comparing them to a set of prototypic or exemplary paths." Kockelman relies on notions of prototype and exemplar to break down the division between instrumental and existential valuation. This is pertinent to my argument when we read that the paths that people take or the choices they make depend on the way they map their values. Kockelman notes, "And part of the issue is to be able to articulate where the values came from, historically, or why we should follow them, rationally. Stereotypically, this may involve disclosing values in a public setting, arguing for them, and communicating such values and arguments to others." When Masterani told me that her lover should recognize what's in her heart, or when hijras expected their lovers to be with them at the cost of material gifts, benefits, or profit, they were articulating a desire for recognition of a certain valuation that

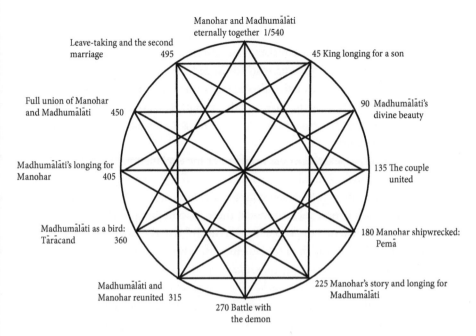

Manohar and Madhumālati
eternally together 1/540

Leave-taking and the second
marriage   495

45 King longing for a son

Full union of Manohar
and Madhumālati   450

90 Madhumālati's
divine beauty

Madhumālati's longing for
Manohar   405

135 The couple
united

Madhumālati as a bird:
Tāracand   360

180 Manohar shipwrecked:
Pemā

Madhumālati and
Manohar reunited 315

225 Manohar's story and longing for
Madhumālati

270 Battle with
the demon

Manjhan's cosmology

they were giving to the men and were expecting in return. The recognition
of that form of valuation would entail following a map that would take
them elsewhere—in the words of Sufi poetry, to paradise—rather than this
world, where social relations are translated (read measured) in propertied
terms.[74]

This was the reason lovers who would not rise to the challenge of taking
on the path of love were often lied to, tricked into fucking, and cheated on,
because in their choosing of material benefits they revealed themselves as
men who were concerned with profit and had failed to recognize the value
of the love that hijras offered. Hijras, in their constant preoccupation with
lovers and love affairs, were holding out the possibility that somebody would
recognize the value of their valuation—one that was different from that
which the world had imposed on the poor, illiterate youths of rural Odisha.
Let us return to Weightman and Hardt to clarify the point of loving cease-
lessly. Weightman argues that each of the six levels of the narrative symmetry corresponds to the six "levels of manifestation of the Absolute"
(see accompanying figure); "the first world, called the *Martaba al-Ahadiyat*,

or the Level of Oneness, is beyond all attribution and determination." I highlight this to reiterate the similarity between the world that can be made possible through love that resists translation into material wealth, as argued by Hardt, and the Sufis who transcend the material world. I argue that hijras in their love affairs also signal toward the shadows of paradise that they feel on this earth, the world that can be, and even though they are cursed to fail at this attempt because catching a mosquito is impossible, they don't give up.

During my research, people would offer me explanations as to why hijras fuck so much. A man who worked at an NGO in Bolongir told me in 2009, ponderingly, "There is something in the sun's heat/ray (*dhup*) in Bolongir that makes people fuck so much; there is something in the *climate* of Bolongir that just makes people fuck so much." Another man who worked in another NGO in Bhadrak told me in 2013, "Hijras have too much *sexual*, that's why they are constantly fucking, no matter how they are feeling—sick or well, they always want to fuck." The words "climate" and "sexual" were used in English and were versions of climatic or constitutional understandings of the relentlessly fucking hijras. Against those two explanations I offer another reading: that of a quest to catch a mosquito, a lover; an attempt to remake one's world that transcends this one—a world that is beyond attribution and determination. The relentless fucking of hijras might keep their flesh weird, like Darger's heroines, and it can be argued that it is similar to the weird flesh that accompanies any spiritual exercise. There might be no evidence for success in these impossible pursuits, but that might be because the story hasn't ended, the grand design is still unfolding; failures are just junctures or points in the journey that one undertakes to achieve the impossible. But like any other shadow, the shadow of paradise may not be sharp or clear in its lines, but its features are still palpable enough to convince one to keep on trying for the impossible, persisting in the pursuit of love.

5

I HAVE IMMORTAL LONGINGS IN ME

This chapter is offered in lieu of a conclusion because many of the questions, concerns, and topics raised are meant to invite further thought rather than resolutions. As the introduction mentioned, HIV should be seen as a watermark that is always there in the background, unquestionably, since hijras have been framed as a high-risk population and a site of at least thirty years of targeted interventions aimed at disseminating HIV prevention mechanisms or "positive living." A watermark allows us to see how the everyday and ordinary struggles of surviving and thriving in the context of poverty were conducted in the shadow of illness and disease—making health a fragile status to maintain or a complex and complicated social endeavor.[1] Many of my friends whose stories and lives I present in this book have now died because of AIDS-related complications; some were only in their twenties or thirties. I have written elsewhere about how the epidemic has colored my life; hence this research. For me the primary goal of studying hijra lives and sexuality was to learn about how we craft our lives and act on our desires while being strangled by the fear and stigma of this disease.

Presently I would like to loop back to retrace the development of my very specific question regarding HIV and hijras over the last twenty years. In a recent essay I gave this account:

My research interest in the HIV epidemic predated my training in Anthropology. It was sparked by graffiti painted on a wall next to one of the many busy traffic intersections in Calcutta. The year was 1995, and I was around nine years old. The graffiti depicted an exaggerated limp wrist, attached to a man against a green background, and read, "Queenies are not the only ones who get AIDS." It was the first depiction I had ever come across of somebody like me. At the time, I was being mercilessly teased and tormented by everybody for being effeminate, and in a way encountering that image shattered my isolation. I welcomed the company of that cartoonish image, painted not as part of any artistic endeavor but to serve a more functional purpose: to dispel misinformation about HIV transmission. I had enough intelligence at that age to understand the implication that "queenies got AIDS."

Though this was my first encounter with the queenie, it wasn't my first encounter with AIDS. A few months before clapping eyes on the queenie, I had seen a photograph in the local newspaper that showed a lot of young children, younger than I was at that time, wearing signs around their necks that said, "AIDS." Some were wearing signs that said "HIV+." My brother and I were both curious, and he had asked our tutor what it meant. Our tutor said, "I don't know"; my brother persisted by saying, "It was in today's newspaper," and I joined in to describe this photograph. Our tutor shook her head and started correcting our exercises with a foreboding expression that shut us up. Fifteen years later, during my doctoral research, I made an educated guess that the photograph was documenting children under state protection who had tested positive for HIV, and the state was segregating them into a separate orphanage. The graffiti has since been long removed but was an early sign of what was to become of the HIV epidemic juggernaut in India as it was already elsewhere in the world. After more than twenty years, I am still pursuing questions regarding sexuality and HIV; in other words, why queenies get AIDS.[2]

By 2003 the epidemic had already generated concern and gained support for the afflicted and affected population from every quarter of civil society in India. The globalizing discourse of LGBT rights, furthermore, allowed activists in India to begin the conversation with the state on issues of access and rights to healthcare and placing the demand for legal recognition and destigmatization of LGBT sexuality as a necessary condition. This is one of the many ways that the history of the LGBT movement in India differs from that in the Euro-American West, where activism around HIV/AIDS built on existing battles for political emancipation that began pre- and post-Stonewall. In India the LGBT social movement was also the HIV-rights movement. By the mid-1990s the field of global health had already framed us as a high-risk population that had to be necessarily addressed, and the clinical veneer allowed the Indian state to put in place an impressive structure to test and treat us, even if not offering any additional political respite from discrimination and abuse. Cipla, the Indian pharmaceutical company that exploited unexpected loopholes in the Indian patent laws, managed to produce generic ARTs (medications to treat HIV), and the company's ambitions aligned with the Indian state's aspiration for a larger share of free-market profits.[3] The continuing battle against patent rights (TRIPS) and the subsequent Doha Agreement made cheap treatment for HIV available across India and Africa. The epidemic also inaugurated the field of global health in India with generous funding made available through organizations like USAID, the UK Department for International Development (DFID), Elton John AIDS Foundation, and the Bill and Melinda Gates Foundation. These were funding bodies with liberal political values that also supported LGBT rights alongside HIV rights, thus giving further support for queer activists. These forces dovetailed to produce an experience of the epidemic that saved us the trouble of having to militantly "wage war"—as contrasted with the activists in the Euro-American West in the 1980s and 1990s, and with the activists in South Africa who had to go on a hunger strike in the early 2000s to demand free treatment.

As Foucault wrote, "Discourse is not life, its time is not your time."[4] In this concluding reflection I turn to the temporal incongruences that exist between our lives, HIV's life, biopolitical life, and the life that might come after death. In 2004 two friends and I slipped into a dark auditorium in Calcutta at an event held in support of LGBT rights. I cannot remember which organization funded the event, but I do remember that the auditorium was largely empty, with handsome gay men sitting in the front hashing it out with the speakers. We three tried to disappear in the back, a bit embarrassed that we were wearing hijra costumes. A speaker started talking about safe sex (it wasn't known as "safer" sex then) and chanted information about condoms, risks, and testing. By now this information had been disseminated so widely that the choir fell silent, and my friends and I looked at each other, bored. We were used to being fed the same lines by state officials, donors, and good-hearted allies, and would have continued sitting silently except that one of my friends scribbled a note and passed it around. The note read, *"Chude chude buro hoe geche, aabar o purono kasundi ghatche,"* which literally translated means, "We've become old, having fucked so much our whole lives, and again they are shoving that old mustard sauce down our throat." The three of us could not suppress our giggles—even under the disapproving gaze of the handsome gays—and we left the auditorium before the event was over. That scribbled note implied a deeper issue: we knew all about safer-sex practices, but nobody was raising the crucial question: *Why were we not using them?* This opaque aspect of our sexuality, while it was felt by a lot of us, was not articulated by any of us. Probably none of us had the language at the time to articulate it, but even if we could have put this question into words we would not have done so because politically it would have been self-defeating. We would not squander our chance to take on the state by acknowledging that even if the state supported us in delivering all our material demands, we would still be irresponsible citizens and not use condoms. Thus, in 2008, I reached Odisha with the help of the friends who had been with me in the auditorium to figure out why we were not using condoms—hence, why queenies got AIDS.

HIJRAS AND GLOBAL HEALTH

There is a misstep in global-health programs that have sought to promote health as an end goal rather than a means that helps us achieve our aspirations and goals; this misstep is probably one of the reasons for the failure to bring down HIV infections in the world. According to a recent study published in the *Lancet*, the annual incidence of HIV has "stayed relatively constant at about 2.6 million per year" since 2005.[5] These numbers reflect how living with health and sexual desire is produced as incommensurable with each other, as an either/or: either one can act on one's sexual desire or one can have health. They also show that global health reproduces and encourages a normative practice of sexuality. The category of MSM (men who have sex with men) illustrates how stigma is displaced from identities to desires in global-health discourse.

The data from the baseline survey of the Pehchan program, which was run by the organization India HIV/AIDS Alliance, delineates the sexual relationships between women and MSM, transgenders, and the hijra population and gives us an idea of the possible routes by which HIV spreads. The Pehchan program is a consortium of organizations that received support from the Global Fund to address the HIV-prevention needs of two hundred community-based organizations across India, specifically addressing the needs of men who have sex with men (MSM), transgenders, and hijras. The Pehchan data was published in a poster, "Sexual Behaviour of MSM, Transgenders and Hijras with Female Partners: An Analysis of Data from the Baseline Survey of the Global Fund–Supported Pehchan Program in India."[6] The title itself illustrates the ideological underpinnings of global health by focusing on the queerness of the population—MSM, transgenders, and hijras—even when the sexual act studied is heterosexual. It not only confirms the limitation of the homo/hetero binary in that the MSM, transgenders, and hijras are also engaging in heterosexual sex but also that the sexual identities have limited correspondence with sexual desire or practices. The report contains a table, reproduced here (see table), indicating the percentages of various MSM populations that have had a sexual encounter with a female partner. The table reveals that 9 percent of the transgender respondents (hijras are grouped in with transgenders) have had sex with a female partner. The report also states that 13 percent of the TG/hijra respondents were married to women. The data further divides female partners into "regular" and "non-regular" and informs us that the "female partners of MSM are often girlfriends and spouses" to emphasize the point that condom use is low between MSM and their regular female partners.

Let us examine the implications of the difference between these two numbers—the 9 percent of hijras who have had sex with women and the 13 percent who are married to women—against the two different schemes

Ever Had Sex with Any Female Partner (by self-identification)

Ever had sexual encounter	All	Gay	Kothi/ B-MSM/ M'mukhi	Panthi/ A-MSM	DD/ AB-MSM	Bisexual	MSM	TG
Yes	46%	14%	35%	71%	75%	88%	45%	9%
No	48%	10%	61%	27%	22%	9%	53%	82%
No Response	6%	76%	4%	2%	3%	3%	2%	9%
Total	100%	100%	100%	100%	100%	100%	100%	100%
N (All MSM & TG)	2,542	70	1,163	369	296	164	246	234

of categorization: regular versus non-regular, and "girlfriends or spouses" versus unrelated women. To begin, these two categorizations of female partners show two different relationships that exist between hijras and women, some percentage of which may be overlapping. One kind of relationship is sexual—that would describe the relationship of the 9 percent of the TG/hijra population having sex with women. For the 13 percent of TG/hijras interviewed who are married to women, the relationship would be better described as conjugal. A hijra might be married to a woman but not necessarily be sharing a sexual relationship with her wife. The fact that sexual and marital relationships do not completely overlap leads to the question of whether the women with whom hijras are having sex are necessarily their wives—given that there is another pertinent distinction, that of related and unrelated partners. Thus, it would first be accurate to deduce that hijras might be married to women and some of the hijras might be having sex with their wives either regularly or non-regularly. Furthermore, it can also be concluded that some hijras are having sex with women, regularly or non-regularly, who are not conjugally related to them. Thus the axis of temporality (regularly/non-regularly) is not always aligned with the axis of space (conjugal/commercial/unrelated intimacy); rather, these intersect in ways that remain beyond the reach of classificatory ambitions.

Let me turn to specific examples from my fieldwork to show how this economy of sexuality is rendered incalculable. Pawan hijra (featured in chapters 1, 2, and 4 of this study) was once being teased by other hijras for being an impostor because the most powerful love affair she had had in her life was not with a man but with a woman. When I inquired about this love affair, she said:

Look at my life, my parents and brothers beat me every day mercilessly. When I tried to run away and join a hijra household, even they treated me with disgust because I am bald and ugly. Hijras don't respect each other, and hate each other. Look at how they abuse each other calling each other *hijra, maichiya, ranga, gandu*.[7] Once I was visiting Sambalpur [a neighboring district] with some of my friends to perform at a religious festival and I met this sex worker. She didn't abuse me. The whole night we spent talking to each other. My heart was flooded by her kindness, she didn't mind that I was a hijra, I got fucked by men. She fed me dinner with such love. For once, I was not afraid or sad. I told her that I wanted to get married to her. Even she wanted to get married to me. But after a few months we both realized that it was not going to be possible. Neither she nor I have any money. My family beats me for ten rupees; you think they will arrange my marriage? They will tease and abuse me: "Why does a hijra require a woman?" We even had sex but it wasn't like the sex I have with men, which is only lust; this was love. When men touch me, I already know that after they ejaculate they will throw me out, disgusted. Where would we have lived? If we had gotten married, people would have teased her as well. They would say, "Everybody knows you are a whore, now you are trying to be a pious wife?" We still call each other intermittently, and the day I talk to her I feel so light in my heart.

The narrative of intimacy that Pawan hijra offered is striking because it shows us the exceptions in the logic of MSM that result from unpredictable and unexpected intimate encounters. The woman with whom Pawan hijra had sex was not related to her, nor were the encounters regular, but it was—in Pawan hijra's recounting—one of the most intimate encounters possible for both of them. Clear boundaries between the categories of women that hijras have relations with (regular/non-regular, wives/girlfriends) become untenable in the light of desire and force us to question the relevance of such categories to predict condom use.

Let me offer one more example of the malleability of desire and the exceptions that sexual desires create in classificatory schemes—and their implications for understanding condom use. Narayani, a middle-aged hijra who lives in Charampa, a village in Bhadrak, is married to a woman who has another man for her lover. The people of the village know that her wife's children are fathered by this man, a local bigwig, but Narayani insists that the children are hers. I learned of this scandal when another hijra made fun of Narayani while I was speaking to her by asking in passing, "Are you the father of these children?" But even as Narayani said, "Yes, I am," she looked upset and angry. Narayani later told me the children cannot be hers because she could never have sex with a woman, implying that she was born with defective genitalia. She roams around with the children, holding them by the hand or hoisted onto her hip. A younger hijra teased Narayani by saying, "You are neither the father nor the mother of the children." That's when Narayani told me, "I always wanted to be a mother and now my wife has made me a mother." I asked Narayani where she and her wife were getting money for food and milk now that they had a baby. She replied that her wife's father was helping them out. When I asked both of them why they got married, Narayani replied, "My parents died when I was eight years old. I used to dance at traveling theatre groups and my father-in-law saw me and liked me and got his daughter married to me. Because they are also poor, and I didn't ask for anything so he could get her married to me. I told him that I am a hijra, but he insisted, so I got married thinking that god will bless me for lightening this man's burden."

This marriage resulted in realizing the dreams and ambitions of two people unexpectedly: Narayani became a mother through her wife, and her wife's father was relieved of his "burden." To an extent, this marriage remains within the logic of Lévi-Strauss's argument in that a correct exchange of women has taken place between men. Narayani's wife found it possible to live within this marriage with the comfort—and child-conceiving fertility— of a lover. Both Narayani and her wife were HIV-positive, but they both told me that they had never had sex with each other. The unpredictability of desire makes sure that the topography of marriage, sexuality, and gender do not always match up with each other. Yet, in the context of risk for HIV, as in the Pehchan data cited earlier, the flow of the risk is always imagined as unilateral—that is, from the sex outside of marriage to heterosexual conjugality.

Categories proliferate as the epidemic grows. MSM has expanded to include, for example, A-MSM (men who penetrate), B-MSM (men who are penetrated), AB-MSM (men who do both). The categories proliferate because they and their classificatory schemes fail to render the sexual field of any given place in time isomorphic with the epidemiological concerns to gauge risk. Meanwhile, many men in the world have started to claim MSM as an identity, indigenizing what started as a global-health or Western category, much like its earlier variants, homosexual and gay. Tom Boellstorff has not only offered a genealogy of the phrase "MSM" but has also argued that "quests for a 'better term' are doomed to failure because they are based on a logic of enumeration, founded on an impoverished theory of language as having the potential to transparently label reality."[8] The impoverished theory of language is related to an impoverished theory of sexuality, which is often conflated with identity, role, and practice, when desire works in a way that renders sexuality incalculable.[9]

BAREBACKING IN BHADRAK AND BHAWANIPATNA

In the decade spanning my first visit to my field-research sites in 2008 to my last in 2018, we all discovered each other's HIV status. We learned it from gossip, or confidences made in the middle of the night when we were feeling particularly melancholic, which was often. Moreover, the staff members of the NGO and the hospital serving small villages and towns did not keep their mouths shut: the HIV counselor would tell the NGO staff, and the NGO staff would tell our neighbors. Meanwhile, the HIV-prevention programs advertised constantly framed us as potential carriers of disease. The men who would visit us knew as well, so it is not as if it was our sole burden and responsibility to use a condom. One young man told Jaina that he was going to fuck another hijra. Jaina immediately told him, "Look, she has HIV, use a condom." He said, "No, I don't like it and I'm not going to use one." Jaina got angry, roped me in and said, "Look at what he is saying." The young man quickly backed down and said he was not going to fuck that hijra, that he was just joking. With everyday exchanges like this, HIV and AIDS got absorbed into the web of relatedness in the village and into the large swath of poverty-stricken India as well. Unlike the beautiful, rich, white gay men of the epidemic, who were not meant to die in their youth, the poor hijra and her lovers in this corner of the world were the population to "let die."[10] Absent were the metaphors of war that literary gay men used to characterized the loss of their and their friends' lives in the West during the pre-ART days—the only instance when young white men died after WWII—and also absent was the rage or the feeling of injustice at those deaths.[11] Yet this argument raises an old Foucauldian dilemma: biopower works differently at the level of the population than at the level of the person. Even if hijras are allowed to die by the biopolitical state, this does not immediately translate into why we would not use condoms. In other words, the key questions remain to be posed: How were we living with the risk of death that not using condoms entailed? And what was our relationship to dying that not using ART entailed?

Hijras would occasionally talk about their HIV status and living with HIV, and in this book I have sought to follow hijras' sensibility in keeping that discourse veiled precisely to reveal the gap between the rules of global health and the everyday ordinary preoccupations of a high-risk group that made following those rules difficult. This book reflects the concerns that hijras had at the level of the everyday: love, sex, family, money—not HIV/AIDS, condoms, health, and death. Concerns of the everyday triumphed over a future that became more and more uncertain with seroconversion. The experiences of hijras that I have tracked in the preceding chapters show that their lives were more devoted to the aesthetics of living—the flirting in the marketplaces and the fucking in the fields, the participation and modulation of the violence in domestic life, the demand for accountability arising out of a logic of noncruelty in the transactions on the trains, and finally the labor of loving—maybe without optimism, but always with the hope that another world will unfold. "Accusations of illiteracy" and ideas of "condom fatigue" are folded into life and the everyday in unrecognized forms.[12]

But still anxieties about contracting HIV did persist in Odisha, and the discovery of one's HIV status did result in extreme distress—nobody wanted to die from it. The sexuality I am describing is not about fetishizing the virus that marks the subculture of barebacking; rather, it is about not bothering with condoms in the hope that we don't contract HIV.[13] Mangu once dismissed the use of condoms by saying, "When a man is fucking, even if a tiger approaches to kill him, he won't stop having sex, he will first finish then he will see to the tiger—how will he stop to wear a condom?" I have attempted to show what is at stake in hijras' sexuality that would muffle the discourse of the risks of contracting HIV. The pathology of the disease is such that it lends itself to a risk that is never then and there, like a tiger, but later in a future and meshed in a set of relations that is always uncertain.[14] Sex was always in such shortage that one existed in debt to desire, and emancipation from such a debt was the promise of love sought by hijras. HIV would come up when yet another hijra would die of AIDS; but it was never with a note of urgency, but rather with a sense of uncertainty—one that would be punctured with Damru beginning to dance or somebody distracting everybody with tales of passionate attraction. I, too, stopped raising the topic after a few years, since I was not sure I had any answers to why we were dying from a preventable and manageable disease. I once asked Guruma of Jajpur whether, to her knowledge, a lot of hijras had died of AIDS. She replied, "A lot of my *sanghwale* [associates][15] died in the last twenty years; now that I think of it, I know it was because of AIDS, though at that time we thought it was because they were alcoholics, or got TB, or diarrhea." Guruma did not say this with anger or grief but only with a barely discernible tinge of pathos. She didn't say anything more, and I did not know what else to ask. Now, I could read our snippets and silences as of the epidemic being folded into ordinary everyday lives and realities, rather than disrupting them.

Mangu's observation about sex was similar to what Foucault wrote in *The History of Sexuality*: "Sex is worth dying for. . . . And while the deployment of sexuality permits the techniques of power to invest life, the fictitious point of sex, itself marked by that deployment, exerts enough charm on everyone for them to accept hearing the grumble of death within it."[16] Though Foucault was writing before the birth of the epidemic, his words are prescient insofar as the grumblings of death made by the disease and the epidemic via biomedicine were accepted by hijras about whom I have written. Refusing that grumbling would not mean avoiding sex, given the availability of condoms, but it would be a refusal of the possibility of love and living, if not life.[17] Foucault claimed in an interview that what bothers people is not that two boys have sex but that they "wake up the next morning with a smile on their faces . . . hold hands and kiss each other tenderly and thereby affirm their happiness."[18] There is a relationship between sex and love for hijras that I describe here that was not like the stranger intimacy that has been studied by queer theorists (though there was a lot of that in rural Odisha between hijras and the men that traveled through the train stations of these districts). Neither was it the gay love that Foucault is talking about, one that entails tenderness, even though there was a great deal of that, as well. The relationship between sex and love that I have tried to describe is one in which sex is always seeded with love, allowing for beneficial misrecognitions that sustain living, if not life.[19] Leo Bersani, writing about S/M, critiques Foucault's formulation of gay love as desexualizing pleasure and points out that "the most radical function of S/M is not primarily in its exposing the hypocritically denied centrality of erotically stimulating power plays in 'normal' society; it lies rather in its truly shocking revelation that for the sake of that stimulation human beings may be willing to give up even a minimal control over their environment."[20] Through this reading Bersani recovers the sex that Foucault seemed willing to forsake and extends Foucault's argument to make place for fantasies. Bersani writes, "The shadowy figures of the loving child and the daddy he coaxed out of his terrorizing and terrorized castrating identity, figures who may have helped *them*, Foucault's couple, to spend a night of penile oblation."

The following conversation took place in the hut where Jasmine and I lived, and where all the hijras would congregate after our afternoon siestas and before making our way to the various spots alongside the highway that passed through the district of Kalahandi, where hijras would solicit clients for sex work. Pawan hijra was particularly melancholic that early evening after she had returned from the District AIDS Prevention and Control Unit (DAPCU); she wasn't her usual talkative self, whereas Jasmine was as energetic and dramatic as usual, lamenting, complaining, arguing belligerently about how hijra lives were worthless, how the world did not care whether they lived or died—not even one's own family, friends, lovers, and boyfriends cared, and not even God cared whether a hijra lives or dies. The usual tirade took a new turn when Pawan mumbled, partly to herself, "Maybe it will be better after we all die." Jasmine pounced on that statement and started shouting, "How will it be better? Who will light our funeral pyres, how will our souls be set free?" At that point, Pawan hijra, who was lost in her thoughts, looked at us with disbelief and asked with concern, "What are you saying? Our souls will not be set free? Will we become spirits/ghosts?" Jasmine continued screaming, "Of course! Do we have sons who will light our funeral pyres?" To this challenge Pawan hijra offered a solution: "You know that widow [who was also a sex worker, and Pawan hijra's close friend], with the son—I shall marry her before I am about to die, then I shall ask her son to light my funeral pyre." All of us began laughing hysterically at this solution—much to the bewilderment of Pawan hijra, who could not understand why we didn't find the solution ingenious and kept on asking, "Why not? What's wrong?"

Whether we would be allowed in heaven or whether our souls would be set free after death was a topic that would emerge periodically in conversations and would result in intense discussion. I was often puzzled as to why hijras were animated by the question of what would happen to us after death; it was only later that I learned to recognize it as evidence of some reprieve from the fatigue that anxieties about HIV/AIDS had induced in all of us.[21] All of us expected first to become infected by HIV and second to die of AIDS-related complications, even despite the promise of ART. Getting infected seemed like an inevitability; every evening when we would take a break from sex with tricks and lovers, comparing notes on who had fucked whom, a small anxiety would inevitably creep up, not just about getting infected but also about passing the infection, irrespective of whether condoms were used or not. Varsha would say about a man, "Oh, I saw a huge boil on his balls, blood was coming out." Nandita would say, "Look, he fucked me dry [without lube] and when he took it out I saw his foreskin was torn and the condom was full of blood." Damru would say, "Just this morning I noticed I have an ulcer in my mouth." Basanti, while waiting for a client, remarked, "Oh, I forgot the condoms," and before I could say anything she said, "Whatever happens, happens, we'll deal with it then" (*Jo hoga dekha jayega*). The certainty of the condom was dependent on a very specific analytics of blood that never matched with the sheer unruliness of the body, let alone sexuality that rendered the entire skin erotic.

The expert knowledge on HIV transmission became unmoored in everyday life; while a condom might protect us, what about the unexpected eruptions, fissures, tears, and ejaculations? It was precisely this incapacity of expert knowledge to contain risk as experienced by hijras at an individual level that resulted in what is now configured as fatigue. The exhausting and futile endeavor of controlling one's entire skin, both inside and out, has been raised in HIV-prevention workshops over the last two decades, and I noticed the change in the late 2000s when *safe sex* became *safer sex*. Yet this acknowledgment of inevitable risk did little to alleviate the stigma surrounding queer sexuality, let alone the anxieties surrounding sex. Expert knowledge, in its refusal to accommodate or address the erotic skin, and by continuing to emphasize genitals and identities rather than the invitations of desire, not only rendered itself suspect for hijras, but the clinic's door seemed closed to hijras—since the medical gaze continues to distribute risk, blame, and stigma rather than apologies and care. This uneven distribution of risk and blame implied by the epidemiological discourse is what I call *clinical homophobia*.

What exactly then is being labeled by the phrase "MSM, transgenders, and hijras with female partners"? In light of ethnographic and lived everyday realities that show that sexuality, risk, and intimacy combine in unpredictable and incalculable ways, the epidemic continues to use big data to attach blame and stigma on already vulnerable populations, albeit in a clinical language. The category "MSM" was coined to designate men who have sex with men but do not identify as gay, but the phrase runs aground in several contexts and fails to escape the shame and stigma or the social realities of nonheterosexual sexuality. Authors of another study in the *Lancet*, for example, explain that while the cases of HIV transmission globally result primarily from heterosexual sex, MSM have higher rates of HIV infection almost everywhere in the world.[22] The authors argue that this is the case "partly because of inadequate information, denial of resources for prevention services of all sorts, and because heterosexism and homophobia marginalize people and make them less able to adopt preventive techniques, even if they are available."[23] While not discounting such an explanation, I would argue that such a contradiction is also the artefact of faulty categories that do not translate effectively on the ground as they do in the clinic.[24]

Robert Lorway and Shamshad Khan show how the acronym "MSM" came to be grafted onto existing cultural expressions of deviant sexuality and thus actually fails to identify men who have sex with men but do not identify as gay; the term is only taken up by those who already identify as men desiring men sexually through various local identities.[25] If we actually take MSM to reference desire as opposed to identities, then we see that men who have sex with men/hijras/TG also have sex with women. And as the Pehchan data shows, there are also hijras/TG who in some contexts, such as marriage, have sex with women. Even if we were to assume that only the A-MSMs or *panthis* (the men who penetrate) are the men who have sex with women, since their desire revolves around penetration, the A-MSM population could be extended to include millions of men who are fathers and brothers, husbands and sons in South Asia. Isolating "sex with men" in this context reveals the inherent homophobia underlying the clinical language of global health. The contradiction that HIV spreads mostly through heterosexual sex, but the MSM have higher rates of prevalence, is a result of the definitional structure of the MSM that insists on splitting sexuality across hetero/homo lines even when they are mostly coterminous with each other for a large part of the world.

People involved in the global response to the HIV epidemic knew early on that the MSM population was also having sex with women, but they did not or could not imagine a proper response to this gap between practice, identity, and category.[26] Therefore, the phrase "sexual behaviour of MSM, transgenders, and hijras with female partners" inadvertently implies that the risk of HIV emerges from the "men who have sex with men," who endanger their "female partners" and therefore heterosexuality. There is an attempt here to make congruent the worlds of marriage, intimacy, and sexuality, which feminist scholars have long shown to be an oppressive affair.[27] Epidemiological discourse mirrors conservative ideals of marriages and women's sexuality that feminists have rallied against. Strangely, women either can have no sex with their MSM husbands because of the incongruence implied through different sexual orientations or they have a lot, which would explain the high rates of HIV because of heterosexual transmission.

THE PROMISE OF HEALTH

Anxieties about ulcers, boils, tears, fissures, cuts, scrapes, and condoms not being used would be mentioned, then disappear like wisps of smoke. They would disappear because other, more pressing matters—the urgencies that constitute the conditions of poverty—demand attention. Matters such as ensuring there is money to buy dinner for family members at home, an aging mother's medicines, overdue repairs, and so on that constituted the hurly burly of everyday life often prevented anxieties of living and dying to be solely linked to HIV and its prevention.

Regarding a different epidemic, in a different country and at a different moment of time, Randall Packard shows how everyday survival for miners in colonial South Africa refracted risk for contracting tuberculosis to ordinary unavoidable objects, in a seemingly intractable process of extractive global capitalism. He writes:

> In 1910 axial-feed water drills began to be introduced. These emitted a fine spray of water that reduced to some degree the dust produced by the drills. Yet the extensive use of water . . . increased the humidity of the mines. This in turn increased opportunities for the spread of tubercular infection as well as the incidence of heatstroke. It also caused the mineworkers' clothing to become soaked from both perspiration and water. This became a serious health problem once the mineworkers left the mine face to return to the surface. The mineworkers would frequently have to walk several hundred feet up an incline to the foot of the mineshaft, sometimes carrying drills weighing thirty pounds. This further increased their overheated condition. Once they reached the foot of the shaft they had to wait to be hauled to the surface. This could take several hours since in many cases the cages that lowered and raised mineworkers were replaced with skips for raising ore during the day. In order to avoid delays

in switching back and forth from cages to rock haulers, black workers were not hauled back to the surface until the rock was removed.

Packard reminds us that for the poor, achieving and sustaining health has been impossible when risk for disease got attached to everything including shirts, winds, profit, technology, sweat, nutrition, and race. Conditions of poverty imprint themselves onto the HIV epidemic to such an extent that living, dying, and surviving get inextricably woven together and become almost indistinguishable from each other. The edict preached by global health then to practice safe sex or cultivate positive living is impossible because it would have to similarly account for everything to be perfectly placed for transmission to not occur. Thus, returning to my metaphor of watermark, we could argue that hijras show us not only what we say about the world but also how we should say it. It would not be sufficient to just point out that condoms were not used and drug regimens not followed, we would also have to show how such goals were put so far above one's reach.

Angela Garcia problematizes the distinction between accidental and intentional overdose in the context of heroin addiction to propose that we recognize "suicide as a form of life." Following Garcia's provocation not to see suicide as an event, but as a way of negotiating life and living that entails a constant awareness of death and dying, hijras' disenchantment with the promise of ART can also be seen not as resistance to biopower but an experimentation with living and dying. This experimentation took a very specific form in rural India. Hijras, when they learned their HIV diagnoses, were understandably upset with the specter of mortality that suddenly came to the fore, but it was only when they were put on the ART regimen that a discrepancy between the desires and dreams of medicine and those of hijras became apparent. Hijras would begin the regimen of medications, then after a while stop. The DAPCU would call the NGO and inquire as to why the concerned hijra had not come for a refill, then the AIDS counselor would make a home visit, placate, cajole, make them understand the importance of taking the medication continuously. Hijras would then get back on ART and after a year or two get off it, then nothing would convince them to go back on it again. Death did not come immediately but over a year that would be marked by slowly withdrawing from other aspects of social life. Some would move out of their homes and start living in *mazars* or *mandirs*, others would move to small ramshackle huts near the cremation grounds or abandoned one-room buildings near public grounds. The long history of asceticism in South Asia that recognizes this form of withdrawal to die as *samadhi maran* prevented the noncompliance from being too forcefully corrected at this point. The history of asceticism also provides us with hints as to how ART reconfigured life for hijras in a way that made compliance difficult and exiting life worthwhile.

Before diagnosis, life and health were a stable ground that could be worked to craft fantasies of love and ethical positions toward kin and to act on desire; a commitment to ART, while not disallowing this form of being, rendered life and health itself something that would entail active commitment. Such a commitment not only put pressures on what were carefully controlled and calibrated relationships with the larger world, including brothers, sisters, lovers, and fellow hijras, but there was nothing worthwhile to be gained. Rather than being abandoned and face social death at the hands of kin and the state (which scholars have studied), hijras actively exited the scene themselves.[28] This was not done to save their families the ignominy and stigma of letting their own die, though this was an important effect; it was done primarily to avoid an unnecessary confrontation that the burden of care would entail. Even if ART promises to give us health, it does not make it possible for us to trace out a linear unfolding of life, youth, parenthood, old age, and then death; health means that hijras once again march toward death diagonally, since our life does not unfold in such decidedly heteronormative stages.

Let me reiterate the question I am grappling with. While biopower might explain the unequal distribution of illness, health, life, and death across populations and result in the grumble of death, it does not explain our forgoing the use of a condom even when it is in our pocket. And secondly, while sex with all its fantasies and possibilities might allow us to misrecognize the pursuit and promise of a fulfilled desire as love that makes the world go 'round, it is not self-evident why the resultant carnality requires risking one's health and giving up the use of condoms[29]—in other words, what is implied about how the social and the subject "gear into each other" in the scene where the condom and ART remain untouched.[30] Amartya Sen, in his critique of a Rawlsian approach to health, writes, "I have tried to argue for some time now that for many evaluative purposes, the appropriate 'space' is neither that of utilities (as claimed by welfarists), nor that of primary goods (as demanded by Rawls), but that of the substantive freedoms—the capabilities—to choose a life one has reason to value."[31] Sen's invocation of capability brings a new dimension into understandings of health. While healthcare might be provided and health encouraged by the state functioning under notions of social justice, the value of health remains unstable and differentiated because of the unequal distributions of capabilities and opportunities to convert health into something of value.

Thus, if we take health to be a form of insurance that ensures a productive future when it can be pressed into service, then a future marked with a sustained threat of poverty, stigma, harassment, disappointment, and betrayals does not keep us alert to preserve health or life. Furthermore, when sexual pleasures exchanged are seeded with the promise, however false, of love, however brief, then the poor hijra body with her ungenerative sexuality gains value, which far exceeds the value that health promises. Value offers us a hinge, which can be manipulated to allow desire and health to be brought closer together or taken far from each other. The various sites where this book places hijras, such as the marketplace, the family, the state, and their lovers' arms, all point to how fraught the experience of value was for poor hijras in rural Odisha. In this context, the lives I have presented warn us away from delineating a strict separation between love and sex, reality and fantasy, and from reducing sex to genitalia. The labor of their loving reminds us that there are immortal longings in us, worth living and dying for.

ACKNOWLEDGMENTS

Foremost, I would like to thank my teachers Roger Bowen, Veena Das, Aaron Goodfellow, Jane Guyer, Naveeda Khan, Harry Marks, Graham Mooney, Deborah Poole, Pamela Reynolds, Charles Sherry, Ashley Tellis, and Susan White. I would also like to acknowledge the help and support that was offered by all the members of the SAATHII (Solidarity and Action Against the HIV Infection in India) offices in Calcutta and Bhubaneshwar. In addition, I would like to express my gratitude to Pawan Dhall and Amrita Sarkar for the warmth of their decades-long friendship.

I would like to thank the Babli Moitra-Kanti Saraf and the Usha Ramanathan-S. Muralidhar households for their food and hospitality during fieldwork. My friends and colleagues read multiple drafts of my chapters, provided incisive comments, threw dance parties, and listened to me ramble for hours. My gratitude to Khushboo Agarwal Raj, Ghazal Asif Farrukhi, Swayam Bagaria, Mariam Banahi, Dwaipayan Banerjee, Roger Begrich, Hester Betlem, Caroline Block, Andrew Brandel, Lotte Buch-Segal, J. Andrew Bush, Sruti Chaganti, Anila Daulatzai, Mansi Goenka, Anaid Citlali Reyes-Kipp Goodfellow, Serra Hakyemez, Fouad Halbouni, Richard Helman, Laura-Zoe Humphreys, Amrita Ibrahim, Andrew Ivaska, Nrupa Jani, Amy Krauss, Victor Kumar, Robert Lorway, Patricia Madriaga-Villega, Callie Maidhof, Andrew McDowell, Sidharthan Maunaguru, Nick Mueller, Sameena Mulla, Zehra Nabi, Sahar Romani, Sirisha Papineni, Ross Parsons, David Platzer, Bican Polat, Maya Ratnam, Sailen Routray, Sandip Roy, Bishan Samaddar, Megha Sharma Sehdev, Svati Shah, Dhanraj Shetty, Chinar Singh, William Stafford Jr., Sailen Routray, Aditi Saraf, Ishani Saraf, and Pooja Satyogi.

Jacob Copeman, Naveeda Khan, and Todd Meyers made themselves always available to read drafts of talks, essays, and articles, often at unacceptably short notice; their support is a remarkable lesson in large-heartedness. Emily Filler, JoAnn Martin, Ryan Murphy, Dan Rosenberg, Nora Taplin-Kaguru, and Elizabeth Angowski made my year at Earlham College memorable and imparted valuable advice on how to become a good teacher. I want to thank the entire QuTub Project team—Benjamin Daniels, Ranendra Kr. Das, Jishnu Das, Ada Kwan, and Madhukar Pai. Thank you for giving me the chance to be part of a truly interdisciplinary research project and for revealing to me the different facets of my questions and expanding my intellectual horizons. Thank you to the members of Institute for Socio-Economic Research on Development and Democracy (ISERDD)—Rajan, Purshottam, Charu, Gita, Bablu, Anand, Varun, Devender—for reminding me every day of the joy and critical import of ethnographic research. Sohrab Hura generously allowed me to use his photograph for the book cover; choosing one from his large, brilliant corpus was a challenge.

My friends and colleagues at Simon Fraser University and in Vancouver provided support and encouragement in every way possible. I thank Lara Campbell, Aman Chandi, Susan Erikson, Lindsey Freeman, Michael Hathaway, Kat Hunter, Vinay Kamat, Helen Hok-Sze Leung, Jen Marchbank, Cait McKinney, Tiffany Muller Myrdahl, Roberta Neilsen, Coleman Nye, Stacy Leigh Pigg, June Scudeler, Travers, and Habiba Zaman. Various editors in varying capacities—Clara Han, Lissa McCullough, Bhrigupati Singh, and Thomas Lay—worked very hard to help me transform my research into a book, revealing in it a potential that was hidden even to me.

I would like to thank my parents, Sunil and Meena Saria, and my brother and sister-in-law, Prateek and Sweta Saria, for their support; and my niece Aavya Mishti Saria, who brings a lot of joy to everybody around her. My uncles, aunts, and cousins supported me so that I too could escape the cruelties of community, and for that I thank them. A lot of my research informants died during the time between my first visit to the field and the time the book was finished; for them I wish I had some other way of commemorating their lives besides these inadequate words. Family members and friends also died—my uncle Deepak Saraf, whose house was always open to me, my grandmother Sita Saraf, who loved without asking any questions, and Kamlesh Desai, who made a trip to India to visit me when things were particularly tough—memories of their love stand for the conundrum that is kinship. I would also like to thank Gregory Sesek for making apparent to me that the design of my life was still unfolding.

The fieldwork on which this book is based was funded by a grant awarded by the Wenner-Gren Foundation. Part of an earlier draft of chapter 1 was published as "The Pregnant Hijra: Laughter, Dead Babies and Invaluable Love," in *Living and Dying in the Contemporary World: A Compendium*, ed. Veena Das and Clara Han (Oakland: University of California Press, 2016), 83–99.

I would like to thank Veena Das for frankly putting up with quite a lot, for her care, attention, patience, and support, for her endless kindness, generosity, and food, all of which I admittedly have taken for granted. Finally, to Aaron Goodfellow, whose gentleness toward me never wavers—his presence and his lessons heal much for me and my world—I dedicate this book.

NOTES

INTRODUCTION: THAT LIMPID LIQUID WITHIN YOUNG MEN

1. Louis Dumont, *Homo Hierarchicus: The Caste System and Its Implications* (Chicago: University of Chicago Press, 1980), 270.

2. Veena Das and Clara Han, eds., *Living and Dying in the Contemporary World: A Compendium* (Berkeley: University of California Press, 2016).

3. For an encyclopedic cross-cultural study of the concept of third gender, see Gilbert H. Herdt, *Third Sex, Third Gender: Beyond Sexual Dimorphism in Culture and History* (New York: Zone, 1994). Evan B. Towle and Lynn Marie Morgan offer an insightful critique of this impulse to curate, universalize, and then operation-alize the "third gender" in other contexts in "Romancing the Transgender Native: Rethinking the Use of the 'Third Gender' Concept," *GLQ: A Journal of Lesbian and Gay Studies* 8, no. 4 (2002): 469–97.

4. Rudi Bleys, *The Geography of Perversion: Male-to-Male Sexual Behavior Outside the West and the Ethnographic Imagination, 1750–1918* (New York: New York University Press, 1995).

5. Thomas R. Metcalf, *Ideologies of the Raj* (Cambridge: Cambridge University Press, 1997), 125. Furthermore, the propinquity of hijras to various traditions of performance can be seen not only in their participation in continuing events of festivals and rural theater, but also in the terms that are still used to describe the plurality within the hijra population—such as *jankhas, bhand, zenanas,* and similar. Also see Jessica Hinchy, *Governing Gender and Sexuality in Colonial India: The Hijra, c. 1850–1900* (Cambridge: Cambridge University Press, 2019).

6. Laurence W. Preston, "A Right to Exist: Eunuchs and the State in Nineteenth-Century India," *Modern Asian Studies* 21, no. 2 (1987): 371–87.

7. For a sample of this growing body of work that critiques easy translation of various forms of "third gender" people to "transgender," see Vek Lewis, *Crossing Sex and Gender in Latin America* (New York: Palgrave Macmillan, 2010); Tom

Boellstorff et al., "Decolonizing Transgender: A Roundtable Discussion," *Transgender Studies Quarterly* 1, no. 3 (August 2014); Marcia Ochoa, *Queen for a Day: Transformistas, Beauty Queens, and the Performance of Femininity in Venezuela* (Durham, N.C.: Duke University Press, 2014); and Nishant Upadhyay and Sandeep Bakshi, "Translating Queer: Reading Caste, Decolonizing Praxis," in *The Routledge Handbook of Translation, Feminism and Gender*, ed. Luise von Flotow and Hala Kamal (London and New York: Routledge, 2020), 336–44.

8. I have written about the spate of parliamentary and jurisprudential arguments ensuring that the rights of hijras are protected. I have pointed out that this sudden attention bestowed by the Indian state is a canny political calculation to absorb hijras into an agenda of religious nationalism; see Vaibhav Saria, "Begging for Change: Hijras, Law and Nationalism," *Contributions to Indian Sociology* 53, no. 1 (2019): 133–57.

9. Lee Edelman, *No Future: Queer Theory and the Death Drive* (Durham, N.C.: Duke University Press, 2004), 3.

10. An example of this very large library of political thought is Ajay Skaria's "Gandhi's Politics: Liberalism and the Question of the Ashram," *South Atlantic Quarterly* 101, no. 4 (2002): 955–86. See also Hent de Vries and Lawrence E. Sullivan, eds., *Political Theologies: Public Religions in a Post-Secular World* (New York: Fordham University Press, 2006), and Talal Asad, *Formations of the Secular: Christianity, Islam, Modernity* (Stanford, Calif.: Stanford University Press, 2003).

11. I borrow the phrase "ethnographically detained" from Alexander Weheliye, *Habeas Viscus: Racializing Assemblages, Biopolitics, and Black Feminist Theories of the Human* (Durham, N.C.: Duke University Press, 2014). Also, for an exposition of the ways in which concepts get worlded and an illustration of how anthropology labors to undo such worlding, see Bhrigupati Singh, *Poverty and the Quest for Life: Spiritual and Material Striving in Rural India* (Chicago: University of Chicago Press, 2015).

12. Edelman responds to Bersani's question through a reading of Hamlet in which Bersani's question is rendered unanswerable: "What *Hamlet* does not and cannot teach, and what we can never know, is how to escape the will-to-be-taught, the desire for a lesson—a profit, a one—to take the place of the zero; how to allow for *not* saying 'yes' to the imperative of life; how to let the future be by being what lets the future"; see Edelman, "Against Survival: Queerness in a Time That's Out of Joint," *Shakespeare Quarterly* 62, no. 2 (2011): 169.

13. Patrick Olivelle, *Manu's Code of Law: A Critical Edition and Translation of the Manava-Dharmasastra* (Oxford: Oxford University Press, 2004), 197.

14. Robert P. Goldman, "Fathers, Sons and Gurus: Oedipal Conflict in the Sanskrit Epics," *Journal of Indian Philosophy* 6, no. 4 (1978): 377n101.

15. Das, *Structure and Cognition: Aspects of Hindu Caste and Ritual* (Delhi: Oxford University Press, 1977), 45.

16. Robert L. Caserio, Lee Edelman, Judith Halberstam, José Esteban Muñoz, and Tim Dean, "The Antisocial Thesis in Queer Theory," *PMLA* 121, no. 3 (2006): 819–28.

17. Apropos, Lauren Berlant insists on the term "sustain" in its various conjugated forms in her conversation with Lee Edelman. Although she is not speaking of Hindu theology in this context, the fact that this concept cropped up in her dialogue regarding negativity and the social suggests that I am not alone in my suspicion. The function of preserving is delegated to Vishnu, whose thousand names in the *Visnu Sahasranama* would include the task of sustaining; see Berlant and Edelman, *Sex, or the Unbearable* (Durham, N.C.: Duke University Press, 2013).

18. Seducing and having sex with men was often referred to as "eating" them; for example, "I want to eat that handsome man," or "I finally ate that handsome man." I would remind readers that the Latin word for brothel is *lupanar*, or "wolves' lair," and the Latin word *lupa* ("wolf") was slang for a prostitute in ancient Rome. See Pascal Quignard, *Le Sexe et l'Effroi* (Paris: Gallimard, 1994), for an exciting analysis of the relationship between the prostitute and the wolf or sex and terror.

19. Leo Bersani, "Flaubert and Emma Bovary: The Hazards of Literary Fusion," *Novel: A Forum on Fiction* 8, no. 1 (Autumn 1974): 26.

20. Richard Halpern, *Shakespeare's Perfume: Sodomy and Sublimity in the Sonnets, Wilde, Freud, and Lacan* (Philadelphia: University of Pennsylvania Press, 2002), 14.

21. *Batli* was the word used for the rectum in the hijra language; it corresponds neither to rectum nor vagina.

22. Jane Guyer writes, "The logic of the burden-of-wealth seems barely compatible with the brightness-of-beauty, in ways to which the collections amplify and offer precision. But they offer few hints towards a resolution of the 'lightness of life'"; Guyer, "The Burden of Wealth and the Lightness of Life: The Body in Body-Decoration in Southern Cameroon," in *Live in Motion, Indeed: Interdisciplinary Perspectives on Social Change in Honour of Danielle de Lame*, ed. Cristiana Panella (Tervuren: Royal Museum for Central Africa, 2012), 264.

23. E. Valentine Daniel, *Fluid Signs: Being a Person the Tamil Way* (Berkeley: University of California Press, 1984), 125.

24. Ibid., 127. See also Caroline Osella and Filippo Osella, "Vital Exchanges: Land and Persons in Kerala," in *Territory, Soil and Society in South Asia*, ed. Daniela Berti and Giles Tarabout (New Delhi: Manohar, 2009), 203–39.

25. Alain Bottéro writes, "Men have to use this essential substance, a true *aura vitalis*, appropriately and with parsimony, for their reserves unfortunately are not endless: It is up to them to dispose of it with discretion if they want to avoid a premature decrepitude. A complete hygiene programme, an 'economy of semen,'

results from this"; see Bottéro, "Consumption by Semen Loss in India and Elsewhere," *Culture, Medicine and Psychiatry* 15, no. 3 (1991): 308.

26. Lawrence Cohen, "The History of Semen: Notes on a Culture-Bound Syndrome," in *Medicine and the History of the Body*, ed. Yasuo Otsuka, Shizu Sakai, and Shigehisa Kuriyama (Tokyo: Ishiyaki EuroAmerica, 1999), 113–38.

27. Wendy Doniger O'Flaherty, *Women, Androgynes, and Other Mythical Beasts* (Chicago: University of Chicago Press, 1982), 37.

28. Andrea Long Chu and Anastasia Berg, "Wanting Bad Things: Andrea Long Chu responds to Amia Srinivasan," *Point*, https://thepointmag.com /dialogue/wanting-bad-things-andrea-long-chu-responds-amia-srinivasan/.

29. Government of India, National AIDS Control Organization, *Targeted Interventions under NACP III: Operational Guidelines*, vol. 1, *Core High Risk Groups* (October 2007), 452; http://naco.gov.in/NACO/Quick_Links/Publication /NGO__Targeted_Interventions/Operational__Technical_guidelines_and _policies/Targeted_Interventions_Under_NACP_III_-_Volume_I_CORE_HIGH _RISK_GROUPS/; accessed January 13, 2014.

30. Edelman, "Ever After: History, Negativity, and the Social," *South Atlantic Quarterly* 106, no. 3 (2007): 470.

31. Cohen, "Holi in Banaras and the Mahaland of Modernity," *GLQ: A Journal of Lesbian and Gay Studies* 2, no. 4 (1995): 399–424.

32. Ibid., 404.

33. Adam M. Geary, *Antiblack Racism and the AIDS Epidemic: State Intimacies* (New York: Springer, 2014), 53.

34. I borrow the metaphor of the watermark from Veena Das's "Engaging the Life of the Other: Love and Everyday Life," in *Ordinary Ethics: Anthropology, Language, and Action*, ed. Michael Lambek (New York: Fordham University Press, 2010), 376–99.

35. Here I employ information from the 2001 census of India, since information regarding concentration of populations based on religion is not available from the 2011 national census. See "Table C-1: Population by Religious Community Table for Orissa," Government of India, Ministry of Home Affairs, accessed September 5, 2014; http://www.censusindia.gov.in/DigitalLibrary/MFTableSeries.aspx.

36. See Gayatri Reddy's ethnography *With Respect to Sex: Negotiating Hijra Identity in South India*, Worlds of Desire (Chicago: University of Chicago Press, 2005), especially Chapter 5, "'We Are All Musalmans Now': Religious Practice, Positionality, and Hijra/Muslim Identification," which treats the historical conditions for this kind of confusion.

37. Several hijras would tell me that the word "hijra" comes from the Arabic word *hijr*, which means to break, leave, or renounce. I am not sure whether this alleged etymology is historically valid or verifiable, as it seems to be an instance

of rewriting one's history. Though "hijra" is a Hindustani word and other South Asian languages have their own words that translate as hijra (for example, *aravani* in Tamil, *maichiya* in Odia), the word "hijra" is often used interchangeably with other words denoting the "third gender," regardless of the language being spoken.

38. On my arrival in Bhadrak in 2008 I met eight hijras, but by the time I left in 2012 there were fifteen. The hijra guru (*guruma*) in Jajpur told me that in the last thirty years her household had grown from five to twenty-eight members. This increase is not marginal if we take into account the many that the guru claimed had died because of HIV and old age. Though I attempted to press her into stating in terms of numbers, I would always get a vague answer like, "many." Of the "many" hijras who died, I was able to collect from the *guruma* fragments of stories of their lives and accounts of their deaths. The number of hijras in Bhawanipatna also increased between 2009 and 2013. During my first visit I met four hijras; when I left there were twelve. The increase had resulted from the return of many hijras from cities like Nagpur, Indore, and Jamshedpur, where they found the rules and discipline of the traditional hijra households too strict to adhere to.

39. Mark Doty, "The Unwriteable," *Granta* 110 (2010): 7–24.

40. One of the ways this difference has been located, as argued by Richard Halpern, is through the notion of sublimation: "Instead of regarding art as the displacement of sexual aims, [my argument] posits Shakespearean homosexuality as itself a product or effect of the aesthetic"; Halpern, *Shakespeare's Perfume*, 21. Halpern's argument marks an intervention in queer theory that had hitherto limited itself to the task of making visible or recognizing same-sex passion instead of historicizing the subject of desire.

41. For a glimpse of the challenges discovered in attempts at translating clinical sexual discourse for safer-sex information and for the persistence and transformation of those challenges over the years, see the following articles by Stacey Leigh Pigg: "Languages of Sex and AIDS in Nepal: Notes on the Social Production of Commensurability," *Cultural Anthropology* 16, no. 4 (2001): 481–541; "Expecting the Epidemic: A Social History of the Representation of Sexual Risk in Nepal," *Feminist Media Studies* 2, no. 1 (2002): 97–125; "Globalizing the Facts of Life," in *Sex in Development: Science, Sexuality, and Morality in Global Perspective*, ed. Vincanne Adams and Stacey Leigh Pigg (Durham, N.C.: Duke University Press, 2005), 39–66.

42. Lawrence Cohen writes that sexual desire or even same-sex desire was often "unnamed but instantly recognizable 'this'"; see Cohen, "Holi in Banaras and the Mahaland of Modernity," 421.

43. See Serena Nanda, *Neither Man nor Woman: The Hijras of India* (1990; repr. Belmont, Calif.: Wadsworth, 1999), and Reddy, *With Respect to Sex*.

1. A PRODIGIOUS BIRTH OF LOVE

1. Henri Bergson, *Laughter: An Essay on the Meaning of the Comic* (London: Macmillan, 1911), 98; originally published in French in 1900.

2. Since funeral rituals concerned with dead babies or miscarried fetuses require paternal acknowledgment for proper burial, the throwing of the baby into the river (to which both Jaina and Shamsheri frequently referred) can be read as teasingly declaiming the men as moral cowards and failures who have refused to shoulder their responsibilities, threatening them with public shame.

3. Alfred Gell, "On Love," *Anthropology of This Century* 2 (October 2011); http://aotcpress.com/articles/love.

4. Georg Simmel, *Georg Simmel: On Women, Sexuality, and Love*, trans. Guy Oakes (New Haven, Conn.: Yale University Press, 1984), 134.

5. Margaret Trawick, *Notes on Love in a Tamil Family* (Berkeley: University of California Press, 1992), 18.

6. *Maichiya* is the Odia word for "hijra" and can be used interchangeably with it, as it was in my conversations in Odisha.

7. Bronislaw Malinowski, *Sex and Repression in Savage Society*, Routledge Classics (1927; repr. London: Routledge, 2001), 82.

8. Bergson, *Laughter*, 85.

9. Lee Siegel, *Laughing Matters: Comic Tradition in India* (Chicago: University of Chicago Press, 1987), 292.

10. Hijras who cannot afford silicone breast implants take birth control pills to grow breasts, which sometimes results in discharge from their nipples. When hijras lactate it causes a lot of excitement, and it is considered a great event. Both Reddy and Nanda have documented this practice in their ethnographies. When hijras joins hijra households they become a *cela* of the guru of that house. They are given a brass tweezer that is called a *darsan*. *Darsan* also refers to the practice of plucking one's facial hair, which hijras practice rather than shaving, the latter considered very masculine and therefore carrying embarrassing connotations.

11. Lovely belonged to a traditional hijra community where she had been initiated as a *cela* or disciple. The hijra household that Lovely was part of consisted of a hijra guru, her *celas*, and her *nati-cela* (grand disciples).

12. Akhtari is referring to the famous shrine (*dargah*) of Khwaja Garib Nawaz (Benefactor of the Poor), the Sufi saint Moinuddin Chishti (1142–1236), in the northwestern city of Ajmer. There were well-planned bus tours that took people from Bhadrak, in the east, across the subcontinent to Ajmer. A lot of daily talk was about how to raise money for family members who wanted to take these bus tours.

13. This demand for resemblance can be traced back to the laws governing adultery in *Manushashtra*. Doniger writes, "In *The Laws of Manu* there are two

different, conflicting models of paternity, expressed through a single agricul-
tural metaphor: the sower of the seed is the biological father, who may or may not
be the legal husband; the woman is the field, and the owner of the field is the legal
husband. The son born in the field (the wife) by a man other than her legal
husband is known as the *ksetraja* (literally 'born in the [husband's] field,' the
wife's natural son). But there are two ways of looking at this metaphor. The first
assumes that the man who owns the field (i.e., the wife) owns whatever crop is
sown in the field. Manu assumes that the field is entirely neutral, and that the
crop (son) sown in it will always *resemble* the seed (the father). Therefore, you
should never waste your seed by shedding it in another man's 'field'" or wife, but
you are not harmed if another man sheds his seed in your wife (in that you own
the son resulting from that act). Manu thus forbids a man to commit adultery in
another man's wife but encourages him to let a brother produce a levirate heir in
his own wife, through the Indian practice of *niyoga*, in that the widow of a man
who has produced no male heirs is appointed to have a son by that man's younger
brother"; Wendy Doniger, "Begetting on Margin: Adultery and Surrogate
Pseudomarriage in Hinduism," in *From the Margins of Hindu Marriage: Essays on
Gender, Religion, and Culture*, ed. Lindsay Harlan and Paul B. Courtright (New
York: Oxford University Press, 1995), 163 (my emphasis: *resemble*). The hijra
demand for resemblance is then also a demand for the legal proof for paternity.
She is owned by *that* man, and the baby is his (160).

14. Gayatri Reddy, *With Respect to Sex: Negotiating Hijra Identity in South
India* (Chicago: University of Chicago Press, 2005), 134–35.

15. Serena Nanda, *The Hijras of India: Neither Man nor Woman* (1990; repr.
Belmont, Calif.: Wadsworth, 1999), 19.

16. Reddy, *With Respect to Sex*, 135–36.

17. Nanda, *Hijras of India*, 19.

18. I want to signal here the multivalence built into the word *Artha*. It refers to
"wealth" in Thomas Trautmann's translation in *Arthashastra: The Science of Wealth*
(New Delhi: Allen Lane and Penguin Books of India, 2012). Olivelle translates
Artha as "statecraft" (x), "political success" (xvii), as "success" (xxxiii); see Mark
McClish and Patrick Olivelle, *The Arthasastra: Selections from the Classic Indian
Work on Statecraft* (New York: Hackett, 2012). *Artha* is also defined in John
Thompson Platts's dictionary as *arth*, vulg. *arath*, s.m., meaning "object, aim,
purpose, intent; cause, motive, reason, account, sake; interest; advantage, profit,
benefit, use, utility; concern, business, affair, matter; thing; substance, property,
wealth, opulence; worldly prosperity; substance, material, stuff; suit, case" in the
dictionary; John T. Platts, *A Dictionary of Urdu, Classical Hindi, and English*
[1884], digitized ed., http://dsal.uchicago.edu/dictionaries/platts). The proximity of
economy in these definitions with concepts of object, aim, and purpose hopefully
allows me to extend my analysis of a hijra's love as one not having currency. Her

love in reaching fructification twists value into price and currency but also endangers the social and death, then relegates her love back into the realm of noncurrency and purposelessness.

19. N. Hanif, *Biographical Encyclopaedia of Sufis: South Asia* (New Delhi: Sarup and Sons, 2000), 135. The seventeenth-century saint Sultan Bahu (1630–91) has also mentioned *sadaa suhaagan* in at least one of his poems: "Everyone recites the creed of the tongue, few say the creed of the heart / Where the creed of the heart is said, there is no room for the tongue / The lovers say the creed of the heart, what do sophists know? / It is this creed that the master taught us, Bahu, and now I am eternally blessed [*sadaa suhagan*]"; in Sultan Bahu, *Death before Dying: The Sufi Poems of Sultan Bahu*, trans. Jamal J. Elias (Berkeley: University of California Press, 1998), 75

20. Trawick, *Notes on Love*, 186.

21. Siegel, *Laughing Matters*, 225.

22. Ibid., 148.

23. Michael Lambek, "Introduction: Illness and Irony—Recognition and Refusal," in *Illness and Irony: On the Ambiguity of Suffering in Culture*, ed. Michael Lambek and Paul Antze (New York: Berghahn, 2003), 10.

24. Lawrence Cohen, "Senility and Irony's Age," in Lambek and Antze, *Illness and Irony*, 122–34.

25. Clifford Geertz, *The Religion of Java* (Glencoe, Ill.: Free Press of Glencoe, 1960), 242.

26. Aaron Goodfellow, *Gay Fathers, Their Children, and the Making of Kinship* (New York: Fordham University Press, 2015), 76.

27. Sheldon Pollock, "The Social Aesthetic and Sanskrit Literary Theory," *Journal of Indian Philosophy* 29, no. 1 (2001): 197–229, quote on 219–20. The quotes of Pollock that follow are from this text.

28. In Indian aesthetics, laughter (*hasya*) is a coupled or implied emotion (*sthayibhava*) of the accomplished aesthetical and ethical state of *sringara* (love). The way laughter is linked with eroticism gives birth to the particular form or flavor of love that is *sringara*. The eight base emotions (*bhavas*) must be developed with etiquette or rules or be given form through aesthetic accomplishment to give birth to eight flavors (*rasas*), and these eight *bhavas* can be linked to the eight *rasas* (flavors or forms) in three ways—*sthayi, sanchari, satvik*.

29. Amrita is one of many trans women in India who are only partially associated with hijras; these trans women are usually from the cities and work for NGOs that constitute the network of AIDS cosmopolitanism that depends on imparting public-health wisdom to female commercial sex workers, hijras, kothis, and active and passive men who have sex with men. They are a conduit, traveling to and fro between local sites where infection takes place and conferences across the world where global-speak, health, and wisdom are discursive terms, and to

which trans women are invited to gain legitimacy for their concerns. Some do not identify as hijras because of their class and caste differentials, whereas some hijras, on the other hand, are invited precisely because of these differences, which offer legitimacy via their role as local experts.

30. See n. 28.

31. Siegel, *Laughing Matters*, 370.

32. A. C. Bhaktivedanta Swami Prabhupada, trans., *Śrīmad Bhāgavatam: With the Original Sanskrit Text, Its Roman Transliteration, Synonyms, Translation and Elaborate Purports* (Los Angeles: Bhaktivedanta Book Trust, 2011), e-book edition, canto 10, chapter 21, verse 9, p. 2,443.

33. Lawrence Cohen, "Holi in Banares and the *Mahaland* of Modernity," *GLQ: A Journal of Lesbian and Gay Studies* 2 (1995): 399–424; quote on 402.

34. Prabhupada, *Śrīmad Bhāgavatam*, canto 10, chapter 18, verse 6, p. 2,217.

35. Prabhupada, *Śrīmad Bhāgavatam*, canto 12, chapter 4, verse 8, p. 291.

36. Doniger, "Begetting on Margin," 180.

37. This yearning for a child was mutually recognized in each other by hijras and cis women. There was almost an unspoken empathy between them that showed when women in the village had miscarriages and hijras would join the other women in consoling the grieving woman. Women, too, would sometimes joke about hijras' inability to get pregnant, and sometimes they would cluck sympathetically at the cruelty of a god who found it fit to not make hijras mothers. This was a recognition of what Naveeda Khan has called in another context "mutual fatedness." See Naveeda Khan, "Dogs and Humans and What Earth Can Be: Filaments of Muslim Ecological Thought," *HAU: Journal of Ethnographic Theory* 4, no. 3 (2014): 245–64. For a brilliant account of how women would grieve miscarriages that also anchors the similarity between hijras and cis women in their wistful desire for pregnancy and disappointment at its loss, see Sarah Pinto, *Where There Is No Midwife: Birth and Loss in Rural India* (New York: Berghahn, 2008).

38. Siegel, *Laughing Matters*, 5.

2. IN FALSE BROTHERS, EVIL AWAKENS

1. I borrow this notion of a tendency toward tenderness from Freud to frame the calibrations of care that hijras and their brothers undertook toward each other for several reasons. The first is the place of ambivalence that is highlighted in tenderness, which gives the care a predeliberative quality; the second is that this ambivalence also implies the play of multiple temporal arcs. Freud wrote, "The relation of a boy to his father is, as we say, an 'ambivalent' one. In addition to the hate which seeks to get rid of the father as a rival, a measure of tenderness for him is also habitually present"; Sigmund Freud, "Dostoevsky and Parricide," in *The*

Standard Edition of The Complete Psychological Works of Sigmund Freud (1928), ed. James Strachey (London: Hogarth, 1961), 21:4,559.

2. For an introduction to the concept of *karta* in Hindu law, see Ludo Rocher, "'Lawyers' in Classical Hindu Law," *Law and Society Review* (1968): 383–402. For a gendered reading of this concept as it was inherited by the modern Indian state, see Tanika Sarkar, *Hindu Wife, Hindu Nation: Community, Religion, and Cultural Nationalism* (Bloomington: Indiana University Press, 2001), 37–44.

3. To make the numbers clearer, Shamsheri's father had bought twelve *katthas* of land, and each of his three sons, along with their mother, received three *katthas* after his death. The mother's three *katthas* would have gone to her three sons, a *kattha* each. So then in effect Shamsheri's entire inheritance was sold for 53,000 rupees, out of which she paid the maintenance fees of 35,000 to the prostitute-wife. She spent 8,000 on fixing her rented house, buying some goats and chickens. She lent the remaining 8,000 to a neighbor for interest. In all the legal documents that were produced because of the divorce settlement, Shamsheri was not referred to as a hijra with a pronoun of *she*, but as a man with the pronoun *he*. Neither was the affair between Shamsheri's wife and her brother mentioned as the reason for marriage or divorce.

4. Shamsheri is referring to the space provided by law that allows for ownership to be contested on the merit of payments of property taxes in the absence of a title deed or a will.

5. The relationship between land and kinship has its genealogy in several debates that were central to anthropology. The more important of them would be around the question of whether kinship was just a language for economic interests or vice versa; see Edmund Ronald Leach, *Pul Eliya: A Village in Ceylon; A Study of Land Tenure and Kinship* (Cambridge: Cambridge University Press, 1961); and Ward Goodenough, *Property, Kin, and Community on Truk* (New Haven, Conn.: Yale University Press, 1951). For the ambivalence in kinship, see Michael G. Peletz, "Ambivalence in Kinship since the 1940s," in *Relative Values: Reconfiguring Kinship Studies*, ed. Sarah B. Franklin and Susan McKinnon (Durham, N.C.: Duke University Press, 2001), 413–44; and Veena Das and Lori Leonard, "Kinship, Memory, and Time in the Lives of HIV/AIDS Patients in a North American City," in *Ghosts of Memory: Essays on Remembrance and Relatedness*, ed. Janet Carsten (Malden, Mass.: Blackwell, 2007), 194–217.

6. In *Totem and Taboo*, Freud writes, "Sexual desires do not unite men but divide them. Though the brothers had banded together in order to overcome their father, they were all one another's rivals in regard to the women. Each of them would have wished, like his father, to have all the women to himself. The new organization would have collapsed in a struggle of all against all, for none of them was of such overmastering strength as to be able to take on his father's part with success"; Freud, *Totem and Taboo: Some Points of Agreement between the Mental*

Lives of Savages and Neurotics, trans. James Strachey (New York: Norton, 1950), 178–79.

7. Juliet Mitchell offers a more nuanced reading of fratricidal violence implicit in *Totem and Taboo*. Mitchell argues that the archetypal poet "claims that the murder of the primal father was not the work of a group of brothers but the solitary act of the poet himself. This is 'the lie.' History recounts this solitary heroic deed in the epic and then all the other brothers come to identify with the poet-hero. The poet tells his story of derring-do and thereby puts himself as heroic revolutionary killer in the place of the father. Thus, if Freud, along with some nineteenth-century anthropologists, postulates the primacy of a matriarch, then it will not be the father that is being killed and identified with—it will be the triumphant oldest brother"; Mitchell, *Siblings: Sex and Violence* (Cambridge: Polity, 2003), 15–16.

8. Psychoanalytically, it could be argued that these property disputes operate as a mnemonic device that reminds brothers of their capacity and perhaps even predilection toward killing each other.

9. Oliver Mendelsohn, "The Pathology of the Indian Legal System," *Modern Asian Studies* 15, no. 4 (1981). On the importance of locality or residence, he writes, "Rather, problematic social relations have been enlisted to deepen what is basically a conflict over land" (836). This is in reference not just to the physical force, manpower, and coercion over local government officials that the cousins could muster because of their long, continuous residence in the village, but also because of their historical use of the land through residing in the village. See Sylvia Vatuk, "'Family' as a Contested Concept in Early-Nineteenth-Century Madras," in *Unfamiliar Relations: Family and History in South Asia*, ed. Indrani Chatterjee (New Brunswick, N.J.: Rutgers University Press, 2004), 161–92, for an account of how precisely these "problematic social relations" were pressed into service in colonial India to negotiate the imperious attitude that followed the annexations of various principalities.

10. Mendelsohn, "Pathology of the Indian Legal System," 836. I am taking issue with the very neat divide between "family relations" and "socially more distant people" because it is precisely because this divide is never clear that family relations become multiplex. Please see Michael H. Fisher's "Becoming and Making 'Family' in Hindustan," in Chatterjee, *Unfamiliar Relations*, 95–121, for a multiplex account of the family in South Asia.

11. While there are many studies that have analyzed the various components of the Indian legal system, I want to cite Daniela Berti's "Hostile Witnesses, Judicial Interactions and Out-of-Court Narratives in a North Indian District Court," *Contributions to Indian Sociology* 44, no. 3 (2010): 235–63. I do so to give an example of how logics and claims that do not have any legal valence can still affect and define the outcomes of the court. Though the legal system, as Mendelsohn notes,

provides a necessary site to make claims, Berti's case study shows that it can still be manipulated to fit a different standard of legitimacy that is difficult to discern but may appear as pathology or corruption.

12. Ibid., 836–37. This divide between harmony and self-interest is suspect, given that disputes take decades to resolve and the cost of fighting often outweighs the gains; thus, the issue is of claims of legitimacy felt by brothers and, in the case of this chapter, the different set of laws that hijras offer. See Sumit Guha, "The Family Feud as Political Resource in Eighteenth-Century India," in Chatterjee, *Unfamiliar Relations*, 73–95, for the complication of the divide between harmony and self-interest.

13. Juliet Mitchell, in *Siblings*, argues for a focus to be put on lateral relationships (siblings), which according to her argument has been dispensed with for the focus on vertical relationships (parental) in psychoanalysis. I borrow these terms not to mark two different sets of people with whom an ego can and does have relationships but to mark *that relationships themselves change* with the same set of people as time passes and life projects such as marriage and fatherhood are undertaken.

14. Das, "The Act of Witnessing: Violence, Poisonous Knowledge, and Subjectivity," in *Violence and Subjectivity*, ed. Mamphela Ramphele, Arthur Kleinman, Pamela Reynolds, and Veena Das (Berkeley: University of California Press, 2000), 223–24.

15. While Das has used the notion of temporal depths, I have used the notion of temporal arcs. Though there are different implications between the two notions, I am trying to point to one similarity they do share, which is that they make the present polyvalent by suturing the future in different ways. By multiple temporalities I mean the ways in which the memory of the past (of being brothers) is felt to be eroded in the present, thereby allowing the future to be projected as a plausible transformation of a relationship. While Das's use of depth allows her to intimate the span of her informant's marriage, which would go beyond this mortal life to the next, hijras were concerned with the future of the present life.

16. A. K. Ramanujan, "Where Mirrors Are Windows: Toward an Anthology of Reflections," in *The Collected Essays of A. K. Ramanujan*, ed. Vinay Dharwardker (New Delhi and New York: Oxford University Press, 1999), 23.

17. Veena Das, "Masks and Faces: An Essay on Punjabi Kinship," *Contributions to Indian Sociology* 10, no. 1 (1976): 1–10; quote on 5. The legal claims made over property have always been complex in Hindu law. As Imtiaz Ahmad notes, "Hindu law was not traditionally uniform and varied greatly from one part of the country to another. *Mitaksara* law, which prevailed over most of north India, defined coparcenary as a person and his sons and their progeny, but in *Dayabhaga* law there is no coparcenary between a man and his sons even if they live in a single household"; Ahmad, "Between the Ideal and the Real: Gender Relations

within the Indian Joint Family," in *Family and Gender: Changing Values in Germany and India*, ed. Margit Pernau, Imtiaz Ahmad, and Helmut Reifeld (New Delhi and Thousand Oaks, Calif.: Sage, 2003), 44. The difference in Hindu and Muslim law, or the ambiguity in the statutes, would not help hijras escape the claims or the violence of their brothers and siblings who made claims to the land because hijras had no children to whom to bequeath their property.

18. Emily Hudson, *Disorienting Dharma: Ethics and the Aesthetics of Suffering in the Mahabharata* (New York: Oxford University Press, 2013), 209.

19. I am aware that dharma has been studied across disciplines and for centuries and indeed is the crux of the scholarship that deals with the *Mahabharata*. The point that I am making here of dharma is a basic one that differentiates it from morality and ethics, and in fact it subsumes these dichotomies to allow for immoral and unethical actions to be a part of dharma. I borrow this reading from Wendy Doniger, *The Origins of Evil in Hindu Mythology* (Berkeley: University of California Press, 1976), 94–139, and Adam Bowles's *Dharma, Disorder, and the Political in Ancient India: The Apaddharmaparvan of the Mahabharata* (Leiden: Brill Indological Library, 2007), 190–280. Apaddharma refers to dharma that is applicable in times of crisis/emergency.

20. Amarnath Tewary, "India Bihar Families Fight for Sixty-Six Years over a Plot of Land," British Broadcasting Corporation News, May 27, 2013, accessed September 8, 2014, http://www.bbc.co.uk/news/world-asia-india-22479055.

21. Bimal Krishna Matilal, "The Throne: Was Duryodhana Wrong?," in *The Collected Essays of Bimal Krishna Matlial*, vol. 2, *Ethics and Epics* (Oxford: Oxford University Press, 2002), 121.

22. CSL ed., *Mahabharata*, book 5, vol. 1, 27.1, p. 175. canto 27, verse 1. *Mahābhārata: Preparations for War*, book 5, vol. 1, trans. Kathleen Garbutt Clay Sanskrit Library ed. (New York: New York University Press, 2008).

23. Ibid., canto 31, verse 20, 1:222–23.

24. Ibid., canto 55, verse 30, 1:509.

25. Ibid., canto 87, verse 10, 1:17. Vidur was the half-brother of the blind king Dhritarashtra and of Pandu. He was also a reincarnation of Dharma cursed to be born of a *shudra* mother. He was, thus, in some respects the uncle of the Kauravas and the Pandavas. In some retellings of this folktale, Duryodhana said that he would not give to the Pandavas even the amount of land that would fit on a needle's tip, let alone five villages.

26. Das, "Masks and Faces," 14.

27. Lawrence Cohen, *No Aging in India: Alzheimer's, the Bad Family, and Other Modern Things* (Berkeley: University of California Press, 1998), 241.

28. A love that was different from what emerges out of cross-cousin marriage, in which the wives are substitutable, thus being too close or too distant from your brother's wife, is a problem. Different, because Jaina as a hijra could never be the

substitute for any of her brothers. Other hijras who were married to women would often live in a different village, town, or city and would pay periodic visits to their wives. They would always carry the threat of bringing shame to their wives and would negotiate this threat by going in *kadi*. *Kadi* in coded hijra language means to be a man—to wear men's clothes, to walk and talk like a man, and basically not to behave like a hijra.

29. Das, "Masks and Faces," 6.

30. Ibid.

31. Das, "Kama in the Scheme of Purusharthas: The Story of Rama," in *Way of Life, King, Householder, Renouncer: Essays in Honour of Louis Dumont*, ed. T. N. Madan (New Delhi: Motilal Banarsidas, 1982), 200.

32. Das's article "Masks and Faces" has the daughter-in-law being accused of driving a wedge between her husband and his brother; Satinder slapped his own brother "for a mere woman." Daughters-in-law, Das reminds us, can be replaced.

33. My argument is taking forward Veena Das's argument in "Secularism and the Argument from Nature," in *Powers of the Secular Modern: Talal Asad and His Interlocutors*, ed. David Scott and Charles Hirschkind (Stanford, Calif.: Stanford University Press, 2006), 93–112. In her reading of Rousseau, Das sees Sophie's presence as chimerical because she is indispensable for making the individual social, but in doing so also makes him sexed and mortal. Her necessary exclusion allows for the sovereign to give life. In rural Odisha, the brothers would often beat their wives, and I read the fear of the father as the affective emphasis of Das's reading of the relationship between the father/the citizen and the family/the state.

34. "FZS" is a shorthand for kindship relations (Father's Sister's Son) commonly used in anthropology.

35. Kath Weston, *Families We Choose: Lesbians, Gays, Kinship* (New York: Columbia University Press, 1991), 117.

36. Bimal Krishna Matilal writes, "The victorious King Yudhisthira suffered from a supreme depression after the war. Finally, when he decided to give up the throne, and to go on his last journey, called the Mahaprasthan, it was even difficult to find a successor to the throne. For even the five sons of the five Pandavas had been killed. Abhimanyu, son of Arjuna, had been killed much earlier. Uttara, the widow of Abhimanyu, gave birth to a dead son (for he was already killed by Asvatthaman's fatal arrow, which by its magic power entered the womb of Uttara) but Krsna revived him. He was called Pariksita. Thus he was the chosen successor to the throne, which Yudhishthira left behind. And thus ended the great rivalry between the two sides of the royal family, the Kauravas and the Pandavas"; Matilal, "The Throne: Was Duryodhana Wrong?," in *The Collected Essays of Bimal Krishna Matlial*, vol. 2, *Ethics and Epics* (Oxford: Oxford University Press, 2002), 120.

37. This obviously has echoes of what in the anthropological canon was studied under classificatory kinship and group marriage.

38. Leo Bersani, "Father Knows Best," *Raritan: A Quarterly Review* 29, no. 4 (2010): 103–4.

39. Cohen, "No Aging in India," 277.

40. *Bhagvata Purana*, canto 7, chapter 14, line 9, p. 1841.

41. Paul Kockelman writes, "The *self as temporality of semiosis* is essentially the temporality of semiosis understood from the signer's point of view: one's commitments and entitlements to signify and interpret at any moment in one's life and across all moments of one's life. In particular, as a sign event may be understood as establishing a *present*, with a past and future, a signer may be understood as establishing a *presence*, with a history and fate. Indeed, the life, biography or *bios* of a signer may be understood as the chaining together of such presences (into a finite length), which itself is located between two absences (of infinite extent)"; Kockelman, "From Status to Contract Revisited: Value, Temporality, Circulation and Subjectivity," *Anthropological Theory* 7 (2007): 151–76; quote on 168.

42. Mangu works very hard; she is also the most experienced hijra in terms of begging on the trains, since she has been begging since she was fifteen years old. Thirty years of begging have made her bold and brassy, and she manages to procure at least 200 rupees on each train by coercing, cajoling, teasing, and tormenting the male passengers. This makes her also the most favored companion with whom the other hijras want to go begging on trains. In theory, she could earn 24,000 rupees every month just from begging, but there are days when she is very unwell and the weather particularly inclement; thus she manages to earn 8,000 rupees monthly. Madhubabu Pension Yojana gives her 200 rupees per month, and the local NGO gives her 4,000 per month for her work of distributing condoms. She also has two ducks, five geese, and two hens, the eggs of which she sells for another 1,000 rupees. She also sells cowdung cakes at one rupee a piece when she buys them wholesale at three cakes for one rupee, resulting in a profit of 300 rupees. She also goes dancing at festivals, which will earn her another 1,000 rupees in the coming monsoon season. During the wedding season, during the winter, she earns almost 800 rupees per wedding. Mangu also goes to *jatra* (open-air theaters) in Chandbali to solicit customers in the spring, which gives almost 2,000 rupees every spring. In the last month of September during the Ganesh Puja, Durga Puja festival celebrations, Mangu earned 15,000 rupees in total.

43. Sophie Day, "Threading Time in the Biographies of London Sex Workers," in *Ghosts of Memory: Essays on Remembrance and Relatedness*, ed. Janet Carsten (Oxford: Blackwell, 2007), 185. Day continues, "The term 'snapshot' suggests a distance for, close up, this family could never evoke such nostalgia or longing.

Such a family never had existed, nor could it exist, but in the hugely segregated environment of sex work, pictures of past domesticity and intimacy were significant in orienting women towards a future that would be very different from the constraints of the present" (189).

44. C. Nadia Seremetakis, *The Last Word: Women, Death, and Divination in Inner Mani* (Chicago: University of Chicago Press, 1991).

45. Sigmund Freud, "Mourning and Melancholia" (1917), trans. James Strachey, in *The Standard Edition of the Complete Psychological Works of Sigmund Freud*, ed. James Strachey (London: Hogarth, 1957), 14:245.

46. See Das, "Wittgenstein and Anthropology," *Annual Review of Anthropology* (1998): 171–95. Das argues that anthropology as a discipline allows the pain of the other to mark one.

47. Leo Bersani, *The Freudian Body: Psychoanalysis and Art* (New York: Columbia University Press, 1986), 53.

48. Nandita's husband rode her scooter over the railway tracks and broke it so that Nandita had to shell out 10,000 rupees to get it repaired; the insurance was to pay 5,000 rupees for it, but she was a bit skeptical about the promise of insurance. Dev, her nephew and Damru's boyfriend, had gone to Bhubaneshwar to get the spare part required, got it fixed, running around for it, then wanted the 5,000 rupees for himself. But because Nandita refused to give her bank account information required to get the money sent, Dev was very angry and upset with her. Nandita feared that he would try to withdraw the money already deposited in the bank account. Dev stole her passport-sized photographs and threatened to open a bank account in her name, seemingly so that he could have the 5,000 rupees of insurance sent to that account and acquire the money. But Nandita refused to give any information, fearing that he would transfer the money from her existing account to the new account, then run away with all the money.

49. Judith Butler, *The Psychic Life of Power: Theories in Subjection* (Stanford, Calif.: Stanford University Press, 1997), 134.

INTERLUDE: STANDING AT A SLIGHT ANGLE TO THE UNIVERSE

1. *Gandu* might be translated as "faggots" or "sodomites" and is a common pejorative term used in South Asia for homosexuals who like to be fucked in their ass (*gand*). It is also a term used by hijras to describe other hijras whom they perceive not to be hijras at all but just somebody who likes being fucked; in other words, hijras they saw or felt to be lacking a certain authenticity that could always be located elsewhere, as I will show. *Gandus* are also what, pace Lawrence Cohen, the Indian everyman is forced to become vis-à-vis the political order. Gandus are thus abject subject positions, which offer no representation in the structure, let alone hermeneutics.

2. *Gharanas* are usually translated as "houses," not in the sense of a fixed domicile but in the sense of a lineage/dynasty/tradition. The closest example of using *gharanas* in social organization in South Asia would be the various *gharanas* of musical tradition, in which musicians are initiated and trained in interpretation and rendition of music/singing that is particular to and recognizable as being of that house. Gayatri Reddy translates *gharana* as "house," and that seems to be the closest we can get in English if we want to impart a sense of the belonging and identity that membership in a *gharana* affords.

3. The problem of authenticity belies a deeper problem of classification, which I do not have the space to address here, but for an inkling, please see the lucidly written essay by Vinay Lal, "Not This, Not That: The Hijras of India and the Cultural Politics of Sexuality," *Social Text* (1999): 119–40.

4. Lawrence Cohen, "The Pleasures of Castration: The Postoperative Status of Hijras, Jankhas, and Academics," in *Sexual Nature, Sexual Culture*, ed. Paul R. Abramson and Steven D. Pinkerton (Chicago: University of Chicago Press, 1995), 300.

5. Cohen, "Song for Pushkin," *Daedalus* 136, no. 2 (2007): 105.

6. Michael Carrithers, "The Modern Ascetics of Lanka and the Pattern of Change in Buddhism," *Man* 14, no. 2 (1979): 294–95. *Sangha* usually refers to a community of Hindu, Buddhist, or Jain ascetics, mendicants.

7. Veena Das, "Being Together with Animals: Death, Violence and Noncruelty in Hindu Imagination," in *Living Beings: Perspectives on Interspecies Engagements*, ed. James Staples and Penny Dransart (London: Bloomsbury, 2013), 27.

8. See G. Morris Carstairs, "Hinjra and Jiryan: Two Derivatives of Hindu Attitudes to Sexuality," *British Journal of Medical Psychology* 29, no. 2 (1956): 128–38; *The Twice-Born: A Study of a Community of High-Caste Hindus* (London: Hogarth, 1957); and "'Mother India' of the Intelligentsia: A Reply to Opler's Review," *American Anthropologist* 62 (1960): 504. For Morris E. Opler's review and replies, see Opler, "Review of *The Twice-Born: A Study of a Community of High-Caste Hindus* by G. M. Carstairs," *American Anthropologist* 62 (1959): 140–42; "The Hijara (Hermaphrodites) of India and Indian National Character: A Rejoinder," *American Anthropologist* 62 (1960): 205–11; and "Further Comparative Notes on the Hijara of India," *American Anthropologist* 63 (1961): 1331–32.

9. Wendy Doniger O'Flaherty, *Śiva: The Erotic Ascetic* (Oxford: Oxford University Press, 1981).

10. Doniger O'Flaherty, *Women, Androgynes, and Other Mythical Beasts* (Chicago: University of Chicago Press, 1982), 65–66. Elsewhere in the book Doniger briefly mentions the feminization of asceticism, but not in the context of Shiva: "In popular folklore in India today, it is believed that when a yogi retains his seed, the seed is transformed into milk; 'semen of good quality is rich and viscous, like the cream of unadulterated milk'" (quoted from G. Morris Carstairs'

The Twice-Born [English ed. 1957/American ed. 1958], 83–84). "The yogi actually develops breasts, just as a pregnant woman does when her 'seed' [i.e., menstrual blood] is obstructed. It is also said that the yogi becomes 'pregnant' as his stomach swells with the retained seed. The yogi thus becomes like a productive female when he reverses the flow of his male fluids" (44). I refrain from discussing this passage because Doniger's aim is to show the transsubstantiality of milk, which can transform into either semen or breast milk. Furthermore, given that her ascetics have *amogharetas*, they don't help us understand hijras' asceticism or eroticism, but do help us understand to a certain extent Shiva's transgenderism.

11. Sophie Day, "The Re-emergence of 'Trafficking': Sex Work between Slavery and Freedom," *Journal of the Royal Anthropological Institute* 16, no. 4 (2010): 829.

12. Ibid., 831n21.

13. Ibid., 830. Helen Hok-Sze Leung develops a similar insight between trans as identity and trans as ascetic practice of performers in her study of the film *Farewell My Concubine*. Please see her book *Farewell My Concubine: A Queer Film Classic* (Vancouver: Arsenal Pulp Press, 2010), as well as her essay "Trans on Screen," in *Transgender China*, ed. Howard Chiang (New York: Palgrave Macmillan, 2012), 183–98.

3. SOMETHING ROTTEN IN THE STATE

1. Lawrence Cohen writes that "there are true [*asli*] hijras, and there are false [*nakli*] ones; Cohen, "Song for Pushkin," *Daedalus* (Spring 2007): 105. "The anthropology of hijra life has tended to portray the relation between true hijras (who are intersexed or have had the operation, or have been accepted into the community by a hijra guru) and false hijras (who dress and dance as women but are not a third gender, or have not been accepted into the community) in terms of denunciation. But the border between authentic and inauthentic hijra embodiment, or belonging, is as much an improvisational exercise in creating a form of life under varied conditions of patronage and violence as it is a difference constitutive of sexual ethnicity" (105). Related to denunciations is the haloed economy of *izzat* (respect/honor). See Gayatri Reddy's ethnography *With Respect to Sex: Negotiating Hijra Identity in South India*, Worlds of Desire (Chicago: University of Chicago Press, 2005), for a crucial charting of the economy of honor and shame as it pertains to hijra aspirations and accusations. *Gandu* is a pejorative term, and its use by hijras for each other strips them of all the respectability (*izzat*) accorded by asceticism, ritual practice, and spiritual power and reduces them to their desire for getting fucked.

2. *Challa* is a word from hijras' language, Farsi. The Farsi that hijras speak has nothing in common with the Farsi spoken by speakers of the Persian language and dialects. Hijra Farsi has more in common with the various codeswitching of

communities of sexual minorities across the world. It is not recognized as a dialect or even a subdialect. For more on this, see the extensive work done by the anthropologist Kira Hall on the language of hijras: Hall, "Intertextual Sexuality," *Journal of Linguistic Anthropology* 15, no. 1 (2005): 125–44; "'Unnatural' Gender in Hindi," in *Gender across Languages: The Linguistic Representation of Women and Men*, ed. Marlis Hellinger and Hadumod Bußmann (Amsterdam: John Benjamins, 2002), 133–62; and Lal Zimman and Kira Hall, "Language, Embodiment, and the 'Third Sex,'" in *Language and Identities* (Edinburgh: Edinburgh University Press, 2010), 166–78. For examples of the secret languages used by communities of sexual minorities, I would suggest looking at how scholars have studied Polari; Paul Baker, *Polari: The Lost Language of Gay Men* (London: Routledge, 2003).

3. For an idea of what I mean by the fractured nature of policing and governance, see Rajnarayan Chandavarkar, "Customs of Governance: Colonialism and Democracy in Twentieth-Century India," *Modern Asian Studies* 41, no. 3 (2007): 441–70.

4. I have made this claim on the basis of the brilliant historical work done by Jessica Hinchy in her essay "Obscenity, Moral Contagion and Masculinity: *Hijras* in Public Space in Colonial North India," *Asian Studies Review* 38, no. 2 (2014): 274–94. Another influential essay regarding colonial policing and impoverishing of hijra communities is Laurence W. Preston's "A Right to Exist: Eunuchs and the State in Nineteenth-Century India," *Modern Asian Studies* 21, no. 2 (1987): 371–87.

5. Maria Heim, "*Dana* as a Moral Category," in *Indian Ethics: Classical Traditions and Contemporary Challenges*, ed. Purushottama Bilimoria, Joseph Prabhu, and Renuka M. Sharma (Burlington, Vt.: Ashgate, 2007), 191.

6. Jonathan Parry, "On the Moral Perils of Exchange," in *Money and the Morality of Exchange*, ed. Jonathan Parry and Maurice Bloch (Cambridge: Cambridge University Press, 1989), 68, 66.

7. Ibid., 83.

8. Ibid., 80 and 81.

9. Parry writes, "The root of the problem, however, is that in the real world the professional priest is constrained to retain most of what he receives—and the greater the disproportion between receipts and disbursements the greater the burden of accumulated sin. It is the money and goods, which are siphoned out of the flow of exchange by being retained, which are really barren, and which infect the family fortunes with their evil sterility, 'when you give seventeen annas having taken sixteen, then that is auspicious (*shubha*). From this no shortage will result. But if you do not give (in this way), then there will always be a continual decline"; ibid., 78.

10. Jenny Huberman, "The Dangers of Dalali, the Dangers of Dan," *South Asia: Journal of South Asian Studies* 33, no. 3 (2010): 408n8.

11. Ibid., 401.

12. Ibid., 413–14.

13. Parry, "The Gift, the Indian Gift and the 'Indian Gift,'" *Man* 21, no. 3 (1986): 463.

14. Sarah Pinto, *Where There Is No Midwife: Birth and Loss in Rural India* (New York: Berghahn, 2008), and Parry, *Death in Banaras* (Cambridge: Cambridge University Press, 1994).

15. See Veena Das, *Structure and Cognition: Aspects of Hindu Caste and Ritual,* Chapter 2, "On the Categories Brahman, King and Sanyasi" (Delhi: Oxford University Press, 1977).

16. See Parry, "Ghosts, Greed and Sin: The Occupational Identity of the Benares Funeral Priests," *Man* 15, no. 1 (1980): 88–111.

17. Das, "Language of Sacrifice," *Man* 18, no. 3 (1983): 454.

18. James Staples, "Disguise, Revelation and Copyright: Disassembling the South Indian Leper," *Journal of the Royal Anthropological Institute* 9, no. 2 (June 2003): 299.

19. See Paul Robert Greenough, *Prosperity and Misery in Modern Bengal: The Famine of 1943–1944* (New York: Oxford University Press, 1982), for an account of how the body was displayed during the famine of Bengal in the 1940s. See Das, *Critical Events: An Anthropological Perspective on Contemporary India* (Delhi: Oxford University Press, 1995), for how women displayed their bodies after the Sikh riots in the 1980s, demanding accountability from the state for the violence done to their community. Both accounts result from events of extraordinary violence, which were absent from the accounts of begging and display that I am studying.

20. Staples, "Begging Questions: Leprosy and Alms Collection in Mumbai," in *Livelihoods at the Margins: Surviving the City,* ed. James Staples (Walnut Creek, Calif.: Left Coast, 2007), 175.

21. Michael Carrithers, *The Forest Monks of Sri Lanka: An Anthropological and Historical Study* (Delhi: Oxford University Press, 1983), 282.

22. To clarify the logic of extraction that hijras, viewed as ascetics, practice, it may help to note the manner in which Romila Thapar differentiates brahman, *ksatriya,* and *devatas* (gods) from each other. Thapar writes, "The *brahmana* as priest had a relationship of reciprocity with the *ksatriya* embodying political power. The sacrificial ritual was an exchange in which the gods were the recipients of offerings, *bali,* the priests were the recipients of gifts and fees, *dana* and *daksina,* and the *ksatriya* as the one who orders the ritual was the recipient of the benevolence of the gods and of status and legitimacy among men"; Romila Thapar, "Sacrifice, Surplus, and the Soul," *History of Religions* 33, no. 4 (1994): 312.

23. Carrithers, "Naked Ascetics in Southern Digambar Jainism," *Man* 24, no. 2 (1989): 225.

24. Carrithers, "Naked Ascetics," 227.

25. Das, *Structure and Cognition*, 38.

26. Gayatri Chakravorty Spivak, "Imperative to Re-Imagine the Planet," in *An Aesthetic Education in the Era of Globalization* (Cambridge, Mass.: Harvard University Press, 2012), 341.

27. Ibid., 350.

28. Ibid., 346.

29. Reddy, *With Respect to Sex*, 244n13.

30. Staples, "Begging Questions," 178.

31. Clifford Geertz argues for a similar definition of *haq* in the chapter "Local Knowledge: Fact and Law in Comparative Perspective," in *Local Knowledge: Further Essays in Interpretive Anthropology* (New York: Basic, 1983), 167–231. Geertz further identifies dharma as a concept comparable to *haq* in the context of Bali.

32. "India Eunuchs Turn Tax Collectors," *BBC News*, November 9, 2006, accessed January 30, 2014, http://news.bbc.co.uk/2/hi/6134032.stm.

33. "India Unleashes Eunuchs on Tax Cheats," *USA Today*, November 9, 2006, accessed January 30, 2014, http://usatoday30.usatoday.com/news/offbeat/2006-11-09-eunuchs-taxes_x.htm.

34. The article, though reporting the use of hijras by Citibank, suddenly and without any explanation begins talking about the difficulty landlords face in collecting rent, the implication being that both the bank and the landlord face similar difficulties and hence employ similarly unorthodox methods to get their money. The article then switches topics seamlessly again to talk about the credit economy in India. I am thus reading into the parallel that the article is drawing between cobras and hijras used by landlords and banks, respectively. I reproduce part of the article here:

> The resort to unorthodox collection methods reflects the frustration of business and industry with debt defaulters, bad tenants and the legal system.
>
> . . . Citibank found that even using agents could cause problems. Repo men working on one of the bank's bad loans repossessed the wrong car, giving rise to an expensive out-of-court settlement and bad publicity.
>
> But with hijras, whose stinging barbs guarantee instant compliance, the balance of terror may have shifted decisively in the bank's favor.
>
> Landlords are also resorting to novel ways to look after their interests, particularly the large tracts of real estate in the capital occupied by tenants still paying 1940s rents on leases signed before India gained independence from Britain.

One landlord in the eastern State of Bihar came up with a novel solution to the problem when he engaged a snake charmer to release cobras into the homes of recalcitrant tenants. A colleague of the landlord said: "The charmer defanged the serpents first, but when you discover a cobra in your water closet, you do not wait to find out if it is venomous."

After that, efforts to evict some tenants and persuade the others to pay market rents went smoothly.

The lack of a national identification system and the failure of credit card companies to share information provides a happy hunting ground for artful dodgers.

35. Jon Boone, "Pakistan's Tax Dodgers Pay Up when the Hijra Calls," *The Guardian*, June 8, 2012, accessed January 31, 2014; http://www.theguardian.com /world/2012/jun/08/pakistan-hijra-transgender-tax-collectors. The article also records how begging divides hijra communities in Pakistan, and though there is an offer of respectability given by working for the state, not everybody takes it. It is precisely the logic of extraction that is afforded by shameless begging that the state is utilizing, thus contradicting its own project to make hijras more respectable. I cite the article here to give another glimpse of the intersection between shame and begging that hijras negotiate. The article goes on to record, "'Begging and sex work is not an honorable job,' says Nirma, a thickset 30-year-old wearing heavy eye makeup and a green sari. But she claims to earn up to £20 a customer and is not impressed by the tax collectors' £90 a month salary. Others say the government should find them jobs singing on television shows. Then again, times are tough, Nirma concedes. Another group of hijras has been encroaching on her patch, she says, and customers are turning to the growing number of female prostitutes in Karachi." The report goes on to cite a hijra, called Natasha, who voices the contradiction in this project of respectability. "It's just so demeaning," says Natasha. "It's no different from begging."

36. Jan McGirk, "Army of Eunuchs Set to Clean Up Bombay," *Observer*, December 14, 1997. This report concerns itself with a certain Govinder Ragho Khairnair, a fifty-three-year-old "who fell foul of local political bosses three years ago" and "is recruiting more than 400 castrated males and hermaphrodites from the port's notorious red-light districts": "With their help, he plans to take on the gun-runners, smugglers and property swindlers who offer bribes to public officials. . . . [Khairnair's] improbable army will use shame and public humiliation as its weapons. Eunuchs will surround an offender and shout insults while raising their saris to flash their mutilated genitalia. 'This will be done to those who misuse the law to harass people,' says Khairnair, who was sacked as deputy commissioner on the Bombay Municipal Corporation after running up against the Chief Minister of Maharashtra, Manohar Joshi, and the radical Hindu chauvinist, Bal Thackeray."

37. Imran Khan, "Bihar to Use Eunuchs to Improve Birth Registration," *Indo-Asian News Service*, March 4, 2012, accessed February 2, 2014, http://www .mynews.in/News/bihar_to_use_eunuchs_to_improve_birth_registration _N434777.html. This article reported that, "worried over the lowest birth and death registration figures in Bihar, the state government has decided to engage eunuchs and traditional cremation workers called 'doms' to improve birth and death registration rates in the state." The principal secretary of the Planning and Development Department, Vijay Prakash, goes on record to say, "Eunuchs visiting families on auspicious occasions like births is an age-old tradition. Their visits would be more fruitful, if they can be engaged to improve the birth registration rate in the state." Both hijras and the state officials rely on an ideological past to further justify this move. The official says, "For ages, eunuchs have been known for collecting information about the birth of children in different localities in each village, town and district." Chandni hijra, a leader of the eunuchs, said, "We have suffered a lot for centuries and most of us live in abject poverty. We want restoration of our recognition on the pattern of the Mughal era." The newspaper report clarifies that Chandni was referring to the practice of "eunuchs being used as palace guards by the Mughals."

38. The newspaper article by J. Dey and Bipin Kumar Singh bore the mildly offensive title "Eunuchs May Prove Potency at Border," *Mid Day*, May 10, 2010, accessed February 3, 2014, http://www.mid-day.com/articles/eunuchs-may-prove -potency-at-border/81190. This article reported that the Arunachal Pradesh home minister, Tako Dabi, wrote to the then Union Home Minister P. Chidambaram, in a letter dated February 23, 2010, suggesting that hijra communities "can be put to use to secure Indo-China frontier." He states, "Eunuchs will discharge effective duties along the international border areas if scope is created for them. . . . If engaged in policing and other paramilitary forces, they may do good service." The article continues, "Dabi has suggested that eunuchs can be employed with minimum remuneration. Usually living in poverty and begging for a living, they may prove quite useful to the nation." According to the article, this seems to be a win-win situation because not only will hijras regain their lost historic respect, but the borders of the state will be kept intact. Home Minister Dabi states in his letter that since hijras "do not have any family, their selflessness is borne out of this detachment which sets them apart from other humans." He goes on to assert, "Eunuchs are more nationalist than any other people. They're physically strong and can be gainfully employed for national security"; the "eunuchs are exception- ally fit for national development duties." Dabi mouths the popular belief that hijras are physically very strong; hence, just as the train passengers are helpless in the face of such strength when harassed for money, the Chinese military along the disputed region will be helpless when they attempt to breach the borders of

India. The reproductive impotency of hijras is transformed into exceptionally lethal potency—like a weapon wielded by the army and border patrols. The *New Indian Express* carried the same story and added, "Faced with isolation, poverty and public ridicule, eunuchs, popularly referred to in India, as 'hijras,' often resort to prostitution for economic survival"; Syed Zarir Hussain, "Use Eunuchs as Border Guards: Arunachal Minister," *New Indian Express*, May 11, 2010.

39. Das, "Sexuality, Vulnerability, and the Oddness of the Human," *Borderlands* 9, no. 3 (2010): 14.

40. Das, "Being Together with Animals: Death, Violence and Noncruelty in Hindu Imagination," in *Living Beings: Perspectives on Interspecies Engagements*, ed. James Staples and Penelope Dransart (London: Bloomsbury, 2013), 25.

41. See also Das, "Violence and Nonviolence at the Heart of Hindu Ethics," in *The Oxford Handbook of Religion and Violence*, ed. Michael Jerryson, Mark Juergensmeyer, and Margo Kitts (Oxford: Oxford University Press, 2013), 15–40.

42. Pratap Chakravarty, "'Incorruptible' Eunuch Takes on Political Giants in Indian Polls," *Agence France-Presse*, May 5, 1996. For an analysis of the figure of the hijra politician, see also Gayatri Reddy, "'Men' Who Would Be Kings: Celibacy, Emasculation, and the Re-Production of Hijras in Contemporary Indian Politics," *Social Research: An International Quarterly* 70, no. 1 (2003): 163–200.

43. "Joketantra: The Semiotics of Castration," *Statesman*, March 7, 2000.

44. Lawrence Cohen makes a similar point: "Ordinary eunuchs were revealed as the real leaders in the same movement that revealed ordinary leaders as the real eunuchs. To put it differently, the embodied *sign* of the operation—both as presence (the wound, the scar) and absence (the hijra's 'hole,' her lack of male genitals)—came to have a paradoxical relation to the embodied *effect* of the operation: the modern sovereign's inability to constitute filial relations with ordinary citizens"; Cohen, "Operability: Surgery at the Margins of the State," in *Anthropology in the Margins of the State*, ed. Veena Das and Deborah Poole (Oxford: Oxford University Press, 2004), 185.

45. "Eunuchs Make Ideal Politicians, Says India's First Eunuch Deputy," *Deutsche Presse-Agentur*, March 7, 2000.

46. "'Original Kinnar' Vows to Fight Out 'Political Kinnars,'" *United News of India*, April 15, 2007, accessed on February 7, 2014, http://news.oneindia.in/2007/04/15/original-kinnar-vows-to-fight-out-political-kinnars-1176636836.html.

47. Nitin Yeshwantrao, "Eunuch Is Odd Man Out in Thane Race," *Times of India*, April 15, 2009.

48. Barry Berak, "Katni Journal: A Pox on Politicians; A Eunuch You Can Trust," *New York Times*, January 19, 2001.

49. Jyotsna Singh, "Eunuchs Boosted by Voter Disillusion," *BBC News*, South Asia section, February 14, 2002.

50. Parry, "The 'Crisis of Corruption' and the 'Idea of India': A Worm's Eye View," in *The Morals of Legitimacy: Between Agency and System*, ed. Italo Pardo (Oxford: Berghahn, 2000), 43, 52.

51. Geertz, *Local Knowledge*, 198.

52. Das, "State, Citizenship, and the Urban Poor," in *Citizenship Studies* 15, no. 3–4 (2011): 320.

53. Ibid., 330–31.

54. Georg Simmel, "The Sociology of Sociability," *American Journal of Sociology* 55, no. 3 (November 1949): 260.

55. Thapar, "Genealogical Patterns as Perceptions of the Past," in *Studies in History* 7, no. 1 (1991): 26.

56. Patrick Olivelle, *The Law Code of Manu* (Oxford: Oxford University Press, 2004), 91, chap. 1, verse 85.

57. Ibid., 91, chap. 1, verse 81.

58. Ibid., 205, verse 301.

59. This myth is recorded very briefly by Gayatri Reddy and by Serena Nanda in slightly different versions, respectively, to make different points; in Reddy's ethnography hijras retold this myth to make a point about better times to come, whereas in Nanda's account hijras used the myth to justify the respect they command in India.

60. Sunita Aron, "The Kalyug Rulers," *Hindustan Times*, December 13, 2000.

61. Vyāsa, *The Mahabharata*, vol. 2, bk. 2, *The Book of Assembly*, and bk. 3, *The Book of the Forest*, trans. J. A. B. van Buitenen (Chicago: University of Chicago Press, 1981), 586, 587, 596 (emphasis mine).

62. "Two Railway Officials Attacked by Eunuchs," *Indo-Asian News Service*, November 18, 2011.

63. "Eunuch Held for Killing Live-In Partner," *Indo-Asian News Service*, May 14, 2011.

64. Shashank Shekhari, "Eunuch Gang Leader Killed in Encounter with Noida Police," *Mid Day*, posted on June 8, 2009.

65. Dwaipayan Ghosh, "2 Eunuchs Found Killed, Jewellery and Cash Missing," *Times of India*, October 21, 2009.

66. Rajinder Nagarkoti, "Eunuchs Robbed of Rs 50L," *Times of India*, May 5, 2011.

67. Das, *Structure and Cognition*, 89.

68. Accountability in the discipline of anthropology is in no way a new topic or concern. The possibility I mention previously—that is, that hijras might be perpetuating *kalyug* rather than making life in it bearable—arises from the provoking words of John Borneman: "While memory over time seeks accountability, money over time evades accountability"; Borneman, "On Money and the Memory of Loss," *Etnografica* 6, no. 2 (2002): 288.

1. I don't know the young boy's exact age. The constraints of ethical research did not permit me to make any kind of contact with him. All the information recorded here was heard in the marketplace recounted by the members of the *panchayat*, one of whom was Jaina. I was told that the boy had flunked the final year of high school, so one can safely assume his age to be eighteen, if not older.

2. Lynn Thomas argues that the appearances of the mythical Parasurama make sensible the goings-on of the epics not only for readers, but for the epic's characters themselves by allowing them and us to tap into mythical time of the other yugas. Her investigation of the anachronistic presence of Parasurama, a main character in the *Mahabharata*, asks how we are to understand Parasurama's intervention in the events of the epics, given that they are set far apart and long after his own lifetime. In response she cites three implications of the temporal dissonance that is created by the presence of the immortal axe-wielding *kshatriya* killer in the chronologies of the epics. First, his presence "brings in focus the scale of the massacre about to take place, and suggests that the reasons for it are similar, namely to relieve the earth of her burden of adharmic *ksatriyas*"; second, he is always present "at the critical junctures between *yugas*"; and finally, "Parasurama acts in a clearly demarcated arena, reaches the limits of his task, and then disappears back to the spatial and temporal sidelines, where he will wait until his reappearance at the next *yuganta*"; Thomas, "Parasurama and Time," in *Myth and Mythmaking: Continuous Evolution in Indian Tradition*, ed. Julia Leslie (Surrey: Curzon, 1996), 73, 83–84. Thomas points out that Parasurama is always present at the transition from one epoch to another. For other examples of how myths change to communicate new thoughts and ideologies, see Laurie Patton's *Myth as Argument: The Brhaddevata as Canonical Commentary* (New York: Walter de Gruyter, 1996).

3. Lawrence Cohen, "Lucknow Noir," in *Homophobias: Lust and Loathing Across Time and Space*, ed. David A. B. Murray (Durham, N.C.: Duke University Press, 2009), 162–84; "The Pleasures of Castration: The Postoperative Status of Hijras, Jankhas and Academics," in *Sexual Nature, Sexual Culture*, ed. Paul R. Abramson and Steven D. Pinkerton (Chicago: University of Chicago Press, 2008), 276–304; and "Science, Politics, and Dancing Boys: Propositions and Accounts," *Parallax* 14, no. 3 (2008): 35–47.

4. When we add to the axis of the *gaandu* and the *nawab* the dimension of age, we find proliferations of the *londebaaz* and his secular, globalizing cousin—the pedophile. Pedophilia does not concern itself with consent—its work is to uphold the legal fiction of the child unable to consent to sex before the decided age, and a valid argument can be made of the necessity of this fiction. Nor does the notion of

pedophilia concern itself with being fucked or fucking when culturally both the positions are highly charged with semanticity, erotic and otherwise. I must add that the juridical is being forced to address, amend, and modify the simple equation of "child and sex equals exploitation of a pure victim" in the increasing number of cases where children of the age deemed nonconsensual with respect to sexuality are committing sexual violence. See Saria, "The Ungovernable and Dangerous: Children, Sexuality, and Anthropology," in *The Way We Stretch Toward One Another: Thoughts on Anthropology through the Work of Pamela Reynolds*, ed. Todd Meyers (Bamenda: African Books Collective, 2017), 71–93. Also see Joseph Fischel's *Sex and Harm in the Age of Consent* (Minneapolis: University of Minnesota Press, 2016).

5. Ruth Vanita, from her introduction to *Chocolate and Other Writings on Male Homoeroticism*, by Pandey Bechan Sharma (Durham, N.C.: Duke University Press, 2009), xxix.

6. Ibid., xxx.

7. Ibid., 63, 64.

8. Cohen, "Holi in Banaras and the *Mahaland* of Modernity," in *GLQ: A Journal of Lesbian and Gay Studies* 2, no. 4 (1995): 399–424.

9. Francis Zimmermann, "The Love-Lorn Consumptive: South Asian Ethnography and the Psychosomatic Paradigm," *Anthropologies of Medicine* 7 (1991): 185–95.

10. Pandey Bechan Sharma, "O Beautiful Young Man!," in *Chocolate and Other Writings on Male Homoeroticism*, trans. Ruth Vanita (Durham, N.C.: Duke University Press, 2009), 55–57.

11. Ibid., 64.

12. Cohen, "Holi in Banaras and the *Mahaland* of Modernity," 418.

13. M. D. Vyas and Yogesh Shingala, *The Life Style of Eunuchs* (New Delhi: Anmol, 1987), 39, 45.

14. Gayatri Reddy, *With Respect to Sex: Negotiating Hijra Identity in South India* (Chicago: University of Chicago Press, 2005), 46.

15. Ibid., 203.

16. Ibid.

17. Ibid., 207–8.

18. Ibid., 47.

19. Ibid., 244.

20. Leo Bersani, "Pedagogy and Pederasty," *Raritan* 5, no. 1 (1985): 16–17.

21. Ibid., 20.

22. Michael Moon, *Darger's Resources* (Durham, N.C.: Duke University Press, 2012), ix.

23. Ibid., 77.

24. Ibid., 78.

25. Veena Das, "Reflections on the Social Construction of Adulthood," in *Identity and Adulthood*, ed. Sudhir Kakar (Delhi: Oxford University Press, 1979), 100.

26. Cohen, "Semen, Irony, and Atom Bomb," *Medical Anthropology Quarterly* 11, no. 3 (1997): 301–3; quote on 302; and "The History of Semen: Notes on a Culture-Bound Syndrome," in *Medicine and the History of the Body*, ed. Yasuo Otsuka, Shizu Sakai, and Shigehisa Kuriyama (Tokyo: Ishiyaku EuroAmerica, 1999), 134.

27. Cohen, "Pleasures of Castration," 298.

28. Caroline Osella and Filippo Osella, *Men and Masculinities in South India* (London: Anthem, 2006), 40.

29. Ibid., 69.

30. I am not sure how much of this is stuff of folklore and rumor and how much of it is an actual practice; irrespective of that doubt, the fact remains that a lot of boys remained unmarried until in their thirties, given their poverty, unemployment, and inability to get suitable jobs.

31. Craig Jeffrey, *Timepass: Youth, Class, and the Politics of Waiting in India* (Stanford, Calif.: Stanford University Press, 2010), 11.

32. Ibid., 75. See also Craig Jeffrey, Patricia Jeffery, and Roger Jeffery, *Degrees without Freedom: Education, Masculinities, and Unemployment in North India* (Stanford, Calif.: Stanford University Press, 2008), especially chapter 6, "Muslims' Strategies in an Age of Insecurity," for a portrait of Muslim youth who have faced additional alienation in the face of saffronization taking place in India.

33. Sharma, "In Prison," in *Chocolate and Other Writings on Male Homoeroticism*, trans. Ruth Vanita (Durham, N.C.: Duke University Press, 2009), 70.

34. Moon, *Darger's Resources*, 120.

35. Father's Brother, Mother's Brother, Mother's Sister's Husband, Father's Sister's Husband.

36. Father's Brother's Son, Mother's Brother's Sister, Father's Sister's Son, Mother's Sister's Son.

37. Another essay by Michael Moon explicates the argument he makes in his book *Darger's Resources*; see Moon, "Do You Smoke? Or, Is There Life? After Sex?" in *After Sex? On Writing since Queer Theory*, ed. Janet Halley and Andrew Parker (Durham, N.C.: Duke University Press, 2011), 55–65.

38. Wendy Doniger, "Transformations of Subjectivity and Memory in the *Mahabharata* and the *Ramayana*," in *Self and Self-Transformation in the History of Religions*, ed. David Shulman and Guy G. Stroumsa (Oxford: Oxford University Press, 2002), 67.

39. Ibid., 70.

40. Robert P. Goldman, "Fathers, Sons and Gurus: Oedipal Conflict in the Sanskrit Epics," *Journal of Indian Philosophy* 6, no. 4 (1978): 325–92; quote on 367n16.

41. James L. Fitzgerald, "Bhisma beyond Freud: Bhisma in the *Mahabharata*," in *Gender and Narrative in the Mahabharata*, ed. Simon Brodbeck and Brian Black (New York: Routledge, 2007), 203.

42. Goldman, "Transsexualism, Gender, and Anxiety in Traditional India," *Journal of the American Oriental Society* 113, no. 3 (1993): 374–401; quote on 380.

43. Sir John Woodroffe, *Introduction to Tantra Sastra*, 5th ed. (Madras: Ganesh, 1969), 34, quoted in Lee Siegel and Jayadeva, *Sacred and Profane Dimensions of Love in Indian Traditions as Exemplified in the Gitagovinda of Jayadeva* (Delhi and New York: Oxford University Press, 1978), 116.

44. See Veena Das's "The Uses of Liminality: Society and Cosmos in Hinduism," *Contributions to Indian Sociology* 10, no. 2 (1976): 245–63. Also see Deepak Mehta's "Self-Dissolution, Politics and the Work of Affect: The Life and Death of Sufi Baba," *Borderlands* 9, no. 3 (2010): 1–23.

45. Bharati Agehananda, *The Tantric Tradition* (New York: Anchor, 1970), 171; quoted in Siegel, *Sacred and Profane Dimensions*, 188.

46. Ibid., 188.

47. David Gordon White, *The Kiss of the Yogini: "Tantric Sex" in Its South Asian Context* (Chicago: University of Chicago Press, 2003), 8.

48. Ibid., 11.

49. Ibid., 14–15.

50. Serena Nanda, *Neither Man nor Woman: The Hijras of India* (1990; repr. Belmont, Calif.: Wadsworth, 1999), 93–94.

51. This is a phrase that one of Nanda's informants used to describe the passionate attachments hijras have to their husbands (93).

52. Nanda, *Neither Man nor Woman*, 25.

53. Ibid.

54. Ibid., 25–26.

55. "Patal" refers to the seven regions that exist beneath the earth; it is distinct from hell, where souls are damned.

56. Reddy, *With Respect to Sex*, 180.

57. Ibid., 185.

58. Ibid., 179. The other koti who had sold his kidney in Reddy's *With Respect to Sex* was Avinash, but Reddy does not have an extensive interview with him.

59. Michael Hardt, "For Love or Money," *Cultural Anthropology* 26, no. 4 (2011): 676.

60. Lauren Berlant, "A Properly Political Concept of Love: Three Approaches in Ten Pages," *Cultural Anthropology* 26, no. 4 (2011): 683–84.

61. Ibid., 690.

62. Ibid.

63. Hardt, "For Love or Money," 679.

64. Nanda, *Neither Man nor Woman*, 70.

65. Hardt, "For Love or Money," 680.

66. Cohen, "Love and the Little Line," *Cultural Anthropology* 26, no. 4 (2011): 694.

67. Ibid., 695.

68. Aditya Behl, *Love's Subtle Magic: An Indian Islamic Literary Tradition, 1379–1545* (Oxford: Oxford University Press, 2012), 29.

69. Ibid., 285.

70. Mohammad Habib, "Early Muslim Mysticism," in *Politics and Society during the Early Medieval Period: Collected Works of Professor Mohammad Habib*, ed. A. K. Nizami (New Delhi: People's Publishing House, 1974), 284.

71. Simon Weightman, "The Symmetry of *Madhumalati*," in *Madhumalati: An Indian Sufi Romance*, trans. Aditya Behl (New York: Oxford University Press, 2001), 230.

72. Reddy, *With Respect to Sex*, 201.

73. Nanda, *Neither Man nor Woman*, 78.

74. Paul Kockelman, "Value Is Life under an Interpretation: Existential Commitments, Instrumental Reasons and Disorienting Metaphors," *Anthropological Theory* 10, no. 1–2 (2010): 149–62.

5. I HAVE IMMORTAL LONGINGS IN ME

1. I borrow the metaphor of the watermark from Veena Das's "Engaging the Life of the Other: Love and Everyday Life," in *Ordinary Ethics: Anthropology, Language, and Action*, ed. Michael Lambek (New York: Fordham University Press, 2010), 376-99.

2. Vaibhav Saria, "The Ungovernable and Dangerous: Children, Sexuality, and Anthropology," in *The Way We Stretch Toward One Another: Thoughts on Anthropology through the Work of Pamela Reynolds*, ed. Todd Meyers (Bamenda: African Books Collective, 2018), 71–93.

3. Dwaipayan Banerjee, "Markets and Molecules: A Pharmaceutical Primer from the South," *Medical Anthropology* (July 13, 2016), http://dx.doi.org/10.1080/01459740.2016.1209499. See also Kenneth X. Robbins and John Mcleod, "Cipla's Journey: How a Muslim-Jewish Romance Shaped One of India's Biggest Pharma Firms"; https://www.lzb.lt/en/2017/10/13/ciplas-journey-how-a-muslim-jewish-romance-shaped-one-of-indias-biggest-pharma-firms/. See also Salil Panchal's "YK Hamied: Cipla's Fearless Crusader"; http://www.forbesindia.com/article/leadership-awards-2016/yk-hamied-ciplas-fearless-crusader/44893/1.

4. Michel Foucault, "Politics and the Study of Discourse," in *The Foucault Effect: Studies in Governmentality*, ed. G. Burchell, C. Gordon, and P. Miller (Chicago: University of Chicago Press, 1991), 53–72.

5. GB 2015 HIV Collaborators, "Estimates of Global, Regional, and National Incidence, Prevalence, and Mortality of HIV, 1980–2015: The Global Burden of

Disease Study 2015," *Lancet HIV* 3, no. 8 (2016): e361–87, quote on e361, http://doi.org/10.1016/S2352-3018(16)30087-X.

6. K. Biswas, G. Kumarikunta, A. Biswas, S. Rakesh, S. Mehta, Abhina Aher, and J. Robertson, "Sexual Behaviour of MSM, Transgenders and Hijras with Female Partners: An Analysis of Data from the Baseline Survey of the Global Fund-Supported Pehchan Program in India," poster session presented at the 19th International AIDS Conference, Washington D.C., 2012; retrieved from http://pag.aids2012.org/EPosterHandler.axd?aid=11333.

7. These are various pejoratives for the third gender.

8. T. Boellstorff, "But Do Not Identify as Gay: A Proleptic Genealogy of the MSM Category," *Cultural Anthropology* 26, no. 2 (2011): 287–312, http//doi.org/10.1111/j.1548-1360.2011.01100.x.

9. P. Aggleton, S. A. Bell, and A. Kelly-Hanku, "'Mobile Men with Money': HIV Prevention and the Erasure of Difference," *Global Public Health* 9, no. 3 (2014): 257–70, http://doi.org/10.1080/17441692.2014.889736.

10. Ann Jurecic, *Illness as Narrative* (Pittsburgh: University of Pittsburgh Press, 2012).

11. Tim Dean, *Unlimited Intimacy: Reflections on the Subculture of Barebacking* (Chicago: University of Chicago Press, 2009), 154. See also E. White, ed., *Loss within Loss: Artists in the Age of AIDS* (Madison: University of Wisconsin Press, 2002).

12. See Cohen, "Accusations of Illiteracy and the Medicine of the Organ," *Social Research: An International Quarterly* 78, no. 1 (2011): 123–42; Dean, *Unlimited Intimacy.*

13. Andrew Holleran, *Chronicle of a Plague, Revisited: AIDS and Its Aftermath* (Boston: Da Capo, 2008). See also Dean, "Bareback Time," in *Queer Times, Queer Becomings,* ed. E. L. McCallum and Mikko Tuhkanen (Albany: State University of New York Press, 2011), 75–99.

14. João Biehl shows us how biomedical technologies encroach on intimacies in Biehl and Amy Moran-Thomas, "Symptom: Subjectivities, Social Ills, Technologies," *Annual Review of Anthropology* 38, no. 1 (2009): 267.

15. *Sangha,* a Sanskrit word that literally means association, is used to refer to groups and units of monks and ascetics in Buddhism, Hinduism, and Jainism. *Sanghwale* was the word Guruma used instead of "friend" for fellow hijras who were not *celas* or *nati celas,* hinting at the structure that is common to all communities of ascetics.

16. Michel Foucault, *History of Sexuality: An Introduction,* trans. Robert Hurley (New York: Pantheon, 1978), 156. For another hearing of this grumble of death, from which I borrow my reading, see Aaron Goodfellow, "Pharmaceutical Intimacy: Sex, Death, and Methamphetamine," *Home Cultures* 5, no. 3 (2008): 271–300.

17. For a more heteronormative version of my argument, please see the brilliant essay by Josephine Aho and Vinh-Kim Nguyen, "Neglecting Gender in HIV Prevention and Treatment Programmes: Notes from Experiences in West Africa," in *The Fourth Wave: Violence, Gender, Culture and HIV in the 21st Century*, ed. Jennifer Klot and Vinh-Kim Nguyen (Geneva: UNESCO, 2011). *The authors note that HIV-positive women would drop out of ART programs after they recovered to resume life—that is, to get pregnant, which would result in them developing resistance to the medication.* For the resistance to life that living with HIV entails even with medication, please see the work of Dominik Mattes, who argues that while access to treatment remains a problem for the HIV-positive population, it does not resolve the issue of how to resume life plans and projects in the proximity of death that the epidemic heralds. His analysis takes Nguyen and Aho's argument further; see Mattes, "'I Am Also a Human Being!' Antiretroviral Treatment in Local Moral Worlds," *Anthropology and Medicine* 19, no. 1 (2012): 75–84, and "Caught in Transition: The Struggle to Live a 'Normal' Life with HIV in Tanzania," *Medical Anthropology* 33, no. 4 (2014): 270–87.

18. Michel Foucault, "The Gay Science," *Critical Inquiry* 37, no. 3 (2011): 393.

19. See Leo Bersani, "Sociability and Cruising," *Umbr(a): A Journal of the Unconscious*, Special Issue: *Sameness* 1 (January 2002): 9–23.

20. Bersani, "Foucault, Freud, Fantasy, and Power," *GLQ: A Journal of Lesbian and Gay Studies* 2, no. 1, 2 (January 1995): 21.

21. Lisa Stevenson makes a similar point when her informants tell her that it is not that they are suicidal but that they do not want to live anymore; see Stevenson, *Life beside Itself: Imagining Care in the Canadian Arctic* (Berkeley: University of California Press, 2014).

22. D. Altman, P. Aggleton, M. Williams, T. Kong, V. Reddy, D. Harrad, and R. Parker, "Men Who Have Sex with Men: Stigma and Discrimination," *Lancet* 380 (9839) (2012): 439–45; quote on 443, http://doi.org/10.1016/S0140-6736(12)60920-9.

23. Ibid.

24. M. Thomann, "HIV Vulnerability and the Erasure of Sexual and Gender Diversity in Abidjan, Côte d'Ivoire," *Global Public Health* (2016): 1–16, http://doi.org/10.1080/17441692.2016.1143524.

25. R. Lorway and S. Khan, "Reassembling Epidemiology: Mapping, Monitoring and Making-up People in the Context of HIV Prevention in India," *Social Science and Medicine* 112 (2014): 51–62, http://doi.org/10.1016/j.socscimed.2014.04.034.

26. T. McKay, "From Marginal to Marginalised: The Inclusion of Men Who Have Sex with Men in Global and National AIDS Programmes and Policy," *Global Public Health* (2016): 1–21, http://doi.org/10.1080/17441692.2016.1143523.

27. F. Agnes, "Hindu Conjugality: Transition from Sacrament to Contractual Obligations," in *Redefining Family Law: Essays in Honour of B. Sivaramayya*, ed. Archana Parashar and Amita Dhanda (New Delhi: Routledge, 2008), 236–57.

28. Biehl, *Vita: Life in a Zone of Social Abandonment* (Berkeley: University of California Press, 2013).

29. See Lee Edelman's helpful critique of barebacking ("Ever After: History, Negativity, and the Social," *South Atlantic Quarterly* 106, no. 3 [2007]) and by extension not using a condom as a literalization of the death drive. Since the death drive works at the level of the unconscious, a literal reading of the death drive would be analogous to asking for a literal and material penis to support the notion of the phallus. See also Edelman, "Learning Nothing: Bad Education," *differences* 28, no. 1 (2017): 124–73.

30. Joan Copjec, "Sexual Difference," in *Political Concepts*, https://www .politicalconcepts.org/sexual-difference-joan-copjec/. See also Alfred Schutz, "On Multiple Realities," in his *Collected Papers*, vol. 1, *The Problem of Social Reality* (Dordrecht: Springer, 1962), 207–59.

31. Amartya K. Sen, *Development as Freedom* (Oxford: Oxford University Press, 2001), 74.

REFERENCES

GOVERNMENT PUBLICATIONS

Biswas, K., G. Kumarikunta, A. Biswas, S. Rakesh, S. Mehta, Abhina Aher, and
J. Robertson. "Sexual Behaviour of MSM, Transgenders and Hijras with
Female Partners: An Analysis of Data from the Baseline Survey of the Global
Fund-Supported Pehchan Program in India." Poster session, 19th Interna-
tional AIDS Conference, Washington D.C., 2012. Retrieved from http://pag
.aids2012.org/EPosterHandler.axd?aid=11333.

GB 2015 HIV Collaborators. "Estimates of Global, Regional, and National
Incidence, Prevalence, and Mortality of HIV, 1980–2015: The Global Burden of
Disease Study 2015." *Lancet HIV* 3, no. 8 (2016): e361–87, quote on e361.
http://doi.org/10.1016/S2352-3018(16)30087-X.

Government of India, Ministry of Home Affairs. *Table C-1 Population by
Religious Community Table for Orissa.* New Delhi. http://www.censusindia.gov
.in/DigitalLibrary/MFTableSeries.aspx (accessed September 5, 2014).

Government of India, National AIDS Control Organization. *Targeted Interventions Under NACP III: Operational Guidelines.* Vol. 1, *Core High Risk Groups.*
New Delhi: October 2007.

NEWSPAPER ARTICLES

"Eunuch Held for Killing Live-in Partner." *Indo-Asian News Service*, May 14, 2011.

"Eunuchs Make Ideal Politicians, Says India's First Eunuch Deputy." *Deutsche
Presse-Agentur*, March 7, 2000.

"India Eunuchs Turn Tax Collectors." *BBC News*, November 9, 2006. Accessed
January 30, 2014. http://news.bbc.co.uk/2/hi/6134032.stm.

"India Unleashes Eunuchs on Tax Cheats." *USA Today*, November 9, 2006. Accessed
January 30, 2014. http://usatoday30.usatoday.com/news/offbeat/2006-11-09
-eunuchs-taxes_x.htm.

"Joketantra: The Semiotics of Castration." *Statesman*, March 7, 2000.

"'Original Kinnar' Vows to Fight Out 'Political Kinnars.'" *United News of India*, April 15, 2007. Accessed on February 7, 2014. http://news.oneindia.in/2007/04/15/original-kinnar-vows-to-fight-out-political-kinnars-1176636836.html.

"Two Railway Officials Attacked by Eunuchs." *Indo-Asian News Service*, November 18, 2011.

Aron, Sunita. "The Kalyug Rulers." *Hindustan Times*, December 13, 2000.

Berak, Barry. "Katni Journal: A Pox on Politicians; A Eunuch You Can Trust." *New York Times*, January 19, 2001.

Boone, Jon. "Pakistan's Tax Dodgers Pay Up when the Hijra Calls." *Guardian*, June 8, 2012. Accessed January 31, 2014. http://www.theguardian.com/world/2012/jun/08/pakistan-hijra-transgender-tax-collectors.

Chakravarty, Pratap. "'Incorruptible' Eunuch Takes on Political Giants in Indian Polls." *Agence France-Presse*, May 5, 1996.

Dey, J., and Bipin Kumar Singh. "Eunuchs May Prove Potency at Border." *MidDay*, May 10, 2010. Accessed February 3, 2014; http://www.mid-day.com/articles/eunuchs-may-prove-potency-at-border/81190.

Ghosh, Dwaipayan. "2 Eunuchs Found Killed, Jewellery and Cash Missing." *Times of India*, October 21, 2009.

Hussain, Syed Zarir. "Use Eunuchs as Border Guards: Arunachal Minister." *New Indian Express*, May 11, 2010.

Khan, Imran. "Bihar to Use Eunuchs to Improve Birth Registration." *Indo-Asian News Service*, March 4, 2012.

Kremmer, Christopher. "Gender-Benders Give Debtors Dressing Down to Make Them Pay Up; India's Repo 'Men.'" *Sydney Morning Herald*, June 13, 1997.

McGirk, Jan. "Army of Eunuchs Set to Clean Up Bombay." *Observer*, December 14, 1997.

Nagarkoti, Rajinder. "Eunuchs Robbed of Rs 50L." *Times of India*, May 5, 2011.

Shekhari, Shashank. "Eunuch Gang Leader Killed in Encounter with Noida Police." *MidDay*, June 8, 2009.

Singh, Jyotsna. "Eunuchs Boosted by Voter Disillusion." *BBC News*, South Asia section, February 14, 2002.

Tewary, Amarnath. "India Bihar Families Fight for 66 Years Over a Plot of Land." *BBC News*, May 27, 2013. Accessed September 8, 2014, http://www.bbc.co.uk/news/world-asia-india-22479055.

Yeshwantrao, Nitin. "Eunuch Is Odd Man Out in Thane Race." *Times of India*, April 15, 2009.

SECONDARY SOURCES

Adams, Vincanne, and Stacy Leigh Pigg. *Sex in Development: Science, Sexuality, and Morality in Global Perspective*. Durham, N.C.: Duke University Press, 2005.

Agehananda, Bharati. *The Tantric Tradition*. New York: Anchor, 1970.

Aggleton, P., S. A. Bell, and A. Kelly-Hanku. "'Mobile Men with Money': HIV Prevention and the Erasure of Difference." *Global Public Health* 9, no. 3 (2014): 257–70.

Agnes, F. "Hindu Conjugality: Transition from Sacrament to Contractual Obligations." In *Redefining Family Law: Essays in Honour of B. Sivaramayya*, edited by Archana Parashar and Amita Dhanda, 236–57. New Delhi: Routledge, 2008.

Ahmad, Imtiaz. "Between the Ideal and the Real: Gender Relations within the Indian Joint Family." In *Family and Gender: Changing Values in Germany and India*, edited by Margrit Pernau, Imtiaz Ahmad, and Helmut Reifeld. New Delhi and Thousand Oaks, Calif.: Sage, 2003.

Aho, Josephine, and Vinh-Kim Nguyen. "Neglecting Gender in HIV Prevention and Treatment Programmes: Notes from Experiences in West Africa." In *The Fourth Wave: Violence, Gender, Culture and HIV in the 21st Century*, edited by Jennifer Klot and Vinh-Kim Nguyen. Geneva: UNESCO, 2011.

Altman, D., P. Aggleton, M. Williams, T. Kong, V. Reddy, D. Harrad, and R. Parker. "Men Who Have Sex with Men: Stigma and Discrimination." *Lancet* 380 (9839) (2012): 439–45. http://doi.org/10.1016/S0140-6736(12)60920-9.

Asad, Talal. *Formations of the Secular: Christianity, Islam, Modernity*. Stanford, Calif.: Stanford University Press, 2003.

Bahu, Sultan. *Death Before Dying: The Sufi Poems of Sultan Bahu*. Translated by Jamal J. Elias. Berkeley: University of California Press, 1998.

Baker, Paul. *Polari: The Lost Language of Gay Men*. London: Routledge, 2003.

Banerjee, Dwaipayan. "Markets and Molecules: A Pharmaceutical Primer from the South." *Medical Anthropology* (July 13, 2016). http://dx.doi.org/10.1080/01459740.2016.1209499.

Behl, Aditya. *Love's Subtle Magic: An Indian Islamic Literary Tradition, 1379–1545*. Oxford: Oxford University Press, 2012.

Bergson, Henri. *Laughter: An Essay on the Meaning of the Comic*. London: Macmillan, 1911.

Berlant, Lauren. "A Properly Political Concept of Love: Three Approaches in Ten Pages." *Cultural Anthropology* 26, no. 4 (2011): 683–91.

Berlant, Lauren, and Lee Edelman. *Sex, or the Unbearable*. Durham, N.C.: Duke University Press, 2014.

Bersani, Leo. "Father Knows Best." *Raritan: A Quarterly Review* 29, no. 4 (2010): 92–104.

———. "Flaubert and Emma Bovary: The Hazards of Literary Fusion." *Novel: A Forum on Fiction* 8, no. 1 (Autumn 1974): 16–28.

———. "Foucault, Freud, Fantasy, and Power." *GLQ: A Journal of Lesbian and Gay Studies* 2, no. 1–2 (January 1995): 11–33.

———. *The Freudian Body: Psychoanalysis and Art.* New York: Columbia University Press, 1986.

———. "Pedagogy and Pederasty." *Raritan* 5, no. 1 (1985): 14–21.

———. "Sociability and Cruising." *Umbr(a): A Journal of the Unconscious.* Special Issue: *Sameness* 1 (January 2002): 9–23.

Berti, Daniela. "Hostile Witnesses, Judicial Interactions and Out-of-Court Narratives in a North Indian District Court." *Contributions to Indian Sociology* 44, no. 3 (2010): 235–63.

Bhaktivedanta Swami Prabhupada, A. C. *Śrīmad Bhāgavatam: With the Original Sanskrit Text, Its Roman Transliteration, Synonyms, Translation and Elaborate Purports.* Los Angeles: Bhaktivedanta Book Trust, 1987.

Biehl, João. *Vita: Life in a Zone of Social Abandonment.* Berkeley: University of California Press, 2013.

Biehl, João, and Amy Moran-Thomas. "Symptom: Subjectivities, Social Ills, Technologies." *Annual Review of Anthropology* 38, no. 1 (2009): 267–88.

Bleys, Rudi. *The Geography of Perversion: Male-to-Male Sexual Behaviour Outside the West and the Ethnographic Imagination, 1750–1918.* New York: New York University Press, 1995.

Boellstorff, Tom. "But Do Not Identify as Gay: A Proleptic Genealogy of the MSM Category." *Cultural Anthropology* 26, no. 2 (2011): 287–312.

Boellstorff, Tom, Mauro Cabral, Micha Cárdenas, Trystan Cotten, Eric A. Stanley, Kalaniopua Young, and Aren Z. Aizura. "Decolonizing Transgender: A Roundtable Discussion." *Transgender Studies Quarterly* 1, no. 3 (August 2014): 419–39.

Borneman, John. "On Money and the Memory of Loss." *Etnográfica* 6, no. 2 (2002): 281–302.

Bottéro, Alain. "Consumption by Semen Loss in India and Elsewhere." *Culture, Medicine and Psychiatry* 15, no. 3 (1991): 303–20.

Bowles, Adam. *Dharma, Disorder, and the Political in Ancient India: The Āpaddharmaparvan of the Mahābhārata.* Leiden: Brill, 2007.

Butler, Judith. *The Psychic Life of Power: Theories in Subjection.* Stanford, Calif.: Stanford University Press, 1997.

Carrithers, Michael. *The Forest Monks of Sri Lanka: An Anthropological and Historical Study.* Delhi: Oxford University Press, 1983.

———. "The Modern Ascetics of Lanka and the Pattern of Change in Buddhism." *Man* 14, no. 2 (1979): 294–310.

———. "Naked Ascetics in Southern Digambar Jainism." *Man* 24, no. 2 (1989): 219–35.

Carstairs, G. M. "Hinjra and Jiryan: Two Derivatives of Hindu Attitudes to Sexuality." *British Journal of Medical Psychology* 29, no. 2 (1956): 128–38.

———. "'Mother India' of the Intelligentsia: A Reply to Opler's Review." *American Anthropologist* 62, no. 3 (1960): 504.

———. *The Twice-Born: A Study of a Community of High-Caste Hindus.* Bloomington: Indiana University Press, 1967.

Caserio, Robert L., Lee Edelman, Judith Halberstam, José Esteban Muñoz, and Tim Dean. "The Antisocial Thesis in Queer Theory." *PMLA* (2006): 819–28.

Chandavarkar, Rajnarayan. "Customs of Governance: Colonialism and Democracy in Twentieth-Century India." *Modern Asian Studies* 41, no. 3 (2007): 441–70.

Chatterjee, Indrani, ed. *Unfamiliar Relations: Family and History in South Asia.* New Brunswick, N.J.: Rutgers University Press, 2004.

Cohen, Lawrence. "Accusations of Illiteracy and the Medicine of the Organ." *Social Research: An International Quarterly* 78, no. 1 (2011): 123–42.

———. "The History of Semen: Notes on a Culture-Bound Syndrome." In *Medicine and the History of the Body,* edited by Yasuo Otsuka, Shizu Sakai, and Shigehisa Kuriyama, 113–38. Tokyo: Ishiyaku EuroAmerica, 1999.

———. "Holi in Banaras and the Mahaland of Modernity." *GLQ: A Journal of Lesbian and Gay Studies* 2, no. 4 (1995): 399–424.

———. "Love and the Little Line." *Cultural Anthropology* 26, no. 4 (2011): 692–96.

———. "Lucknow Noir." In *Homophobias: Lust and Loathing across Time and Space,* edited by David A. B. Murray, 162–84. Durham, N.C.: Duke University Press, 2009.

———. *No Aging in India: Alzheimer's, the Bad Family, and Other Modern Things.* Berkeley: University of California Press, 1998.

———. "Operability: Surgery at the Margin of the State." In *Anthropology in the Margins of the State,* edited by Veena Das and Deborah Poole, 165–90. New Delhi: Oxford University Press, 2004.

———. "The Pleasures of Castration: The Postoperative Status of Hijras, Jankhas and Academics." In *Sexual Nature/Sexual Culture,* edited by Paul R. Abramson and Steven D. Pinkerton, 276–304. Chicago: University of Chicago Press, 1995.

———. "Science, Politics, and Dancing Boys: Propositions and Accounts." *Parallax* 14, no. 3 (2008): 35–47.

———. "Semen, Irony, and the Atom Bomb." *Medical Anthropology Quarterly* 11, no. 3 (1997): 301–3.

———. "Senility and Irony's Age." In *Illness and Irony: On the Ambiguity of Suffering in Culture,* edited by Michael Lambek and Paul Antze, 122–34. New York: Berghahn, 2003.

———. "Song for Pushkin." *Daedalus* 136, no. 2 (Spring 2007): 103–15.

Copjec, Joan. "Sexual Difference." In *Political Concepts*. https://www
.politicalconcepts.org/sexual-difference-joan-copjec/.

Daniel, E. Valentine. *Fluid Signs: Being a Person the Tamil Way*. Berkeley:
University of California Press, 1984.

Das, Veena. "The Act of Witnessing: Violence, Poisonous Knowledge, and
Subjectivity." In *Violence and Subjectivity*, edited by Veena Das, Arthur
Kleinman, Mamphela Ramphele, and Pamela Reynolds, 223–24. Berkeley:
University of California Press, 2000.

———. "Being Together with Animals: Death, Violence and Noncruelty in Hindu
Imagination." In *Living Beings: Perspectives on Interspecies Engagements*, edited
by James Staples and Penny Dransart, 17–32. New York: Bloomsbury, 2013.

———. *Critical Events: An Anthropological Perspective on Contemporary India*.
Oxford: Oxford University Press, 1995.

———. "Engaging the Life of the Other: Love and Everyday Life." In *Ordinary
Ethics: Anthropology, Language, and Action*, edited by Michael Lambek,
376–99. New York: Fordham University Press, 2010.

———. "Kama in the Scheme of Purusharthas: The Story of Rama." In *Way of Life:
King, Householder, Renouncer; Essays in Honour of Louis Dumont*, edited by
T. N. Madan. New Delhi: Motilal Banarsidas, 1982.

———. "Masks and Faces: An Essay on Punjabi Kinship." *Contributions to Indian
Sociology* 10, no. 1 (1976): 1–30.

———. "Reflections on the Social Construction of Adulthood." In *Identity and
Adulthood*, edited by Sudhir Kakar. Delhi: Oxford University Press, 1979.

———. "Secularism and the Argument from Nature." In *Powers of the Secular
Modern: Talal Asad and His Interlocutors*, edited by David Scott and Charles
Hirschkind, 93–112. Stanford, Calif.: Stanford University Press, 2006.

———. "Sexuality, Vulnerability, and the Oddness of the Human." *Borderlands
E-Journal: New Spaces in the Humanities* 9, no. 3 (2010): 1–17.

———. "State, Citizenship, and the Urban Poor." *Citizenship Studies* 15, no. 3–4
(2011): 319–33.

———. *Structure and Cognition: Aspects of Hindu Caste and Ritual*. Delhi: Oxford
University Press, 1977.

———. "The Uses of Liminality: Society and Cosmos in Hinduism." *Contributions
to Indian Sociology* 10, no. 2 (1976): 245–63.

———. "Violence and Nonviolence at the Heart of Hindu Ethics." In *The Oxford
Handbook of Religion and Violence*, edited by Michael Jerryson, Mark
Juergensmeyer, and Margo Kitts, 15–40. Oxford: Oxford University Press, 2013.

———. "Wittgenstein and Anthropology." *Annual Review of Anthropology* 27
(1998): 171–95.

Das, Veena, and Clara Han, eds. *Living and Dying in the Contemporary World: A
Compendium*. Oakland: University of California Press, 2016.

Das, Veena, and Lori Leonard. "Kinship, Memory, and Time in the Lives of HIV/ AIDS Patients in a North American City." In *Ghosts of Memory: Essays on Remembrance and Relatedness*, edited by Janet Carsten, 194–217. Malden, Mass.: Blackwell, 2007.

Day, Sophie. "The Re-emergence of 'Trafficking': Sex Work between Slavery and Freedom." *Journal of the Royal Anthropological Institute* 16, no. 4 (2010): 816–34.

———. "Threading Time in the Biographies of London Sex Workers." In *Ghosts of Memory: Essays on Remembrance and Relatedness*, edited by Janet Carsten, 172–93. Malden, Mass.: Blackwell, 2007.

Dean, Tim. "Bareback Time." In *Queer Times, Queer Becomings*, edited by Ellen Lee McCallum and Mikko Tuhkanen. Albany: State University of New York Press, 2011.

———. *Unlimited Intimacy: Reflections on the Subculture of Barebacking.* Chicago: University of Chicago Press, 2009.

de Vries, Hent, and Lawrence E. Sullivan, eds. *Political Theologies: Public Religions in a Post-Secular World.* New York: Fordham University Press, 2006.

Doniger, Wendy. "Begetting on Margin: Adultery and Surrogate Pseudomarriage in Hinduism." In *From the Margins of Hindu Marriage: Essays on Gender, Religion, and Culture*, edited by Lindsay Harlan and Paul B. Courtright, 160–83. New York: Oxford University Press, 1995.

———. *The Origins of Evil in Hindu Mythology.* Berkeley: University of California Press, 1976.

———. "Transformations of Subjectivity and Memory in the *Mahābhārata* and the Rāmāyaṇa." In *Self and Self-Transformation in the History of Religion*, edited by David Shulman and Guy G. Stroumsa, 57–72. Oxford: Oxford University Press, 2002.

Doty, Mark. "The Unwriteable." *Granta* 110 (2010): 7–24.

Dumont, Louis. *Homo Hierarchicus: The Caste System and Its Implications.* Chicago: University of Chicago Press, 1980.

Edelman, Lee. "Against Survival: Queerness in a Time That's Out of Joint." *Shakespeare Quarterly* 62, no. 2 (2011): 148–69.

———. "Ever After: History, Negativity, and the Social." *South Atlantic Quarterly* 106, no. 3 (2007): 469–76.

———. "Learning Nothing: Bad Education." *differences* 28, no. 1 (2017): 124–73.

———. *No Future: Queer Theory and the Death Drive.* Durham, N.C.: Duke University Press, 2004.

Fischel, Joseph J. *Sex and Harm in the Age of Consent.* Minneapolis: University of Minnesota Press, 2016.

Fitzgerald, James L. "Bhisma beyond Freud: Bhisma in the *Mahabharata*." In *Gender and Narrative in the Mahabharata*, edited by Simon Brodbeck and Brian Black. New York: Routledge, 2007.

Foucault, Michel. "The Gay Science." *Critical Inquiry* 37, no. 3 (2011): 385–403.

———. *The History of Sexuality: An Introduction.* Translated by Robert Hurley. New York: Pantheon, 1978.

———. "Politics and the Study of Discourse." In *The Foucault Effect: Studies in Governmentality,* edited by G. Burchell, C. Gordon, and P. Miller, 53–72. Chicago: University of Chicago Press, 1991.

Freud, Sigmund. "Dostoevsky and Parricide." In *The Standard Edition of The Complete Psychological Works of Sigmund Freud* (1928), edited by James Strachey, 21:4,559. London: Hogarth, 1961.

———. "Mourning and Melancholia" (1917). In *The Standard Edition of the Complete Psychological Works of Sigmund Freud,* edited and translated by James Strachey. London: Hogarth, 1957.

———. *Totem and Taboo: Some Points of Agreement between the Mental Lives of Savages and Neurotics.* Translated by James Strachey. New York: Norton, 1950.

Geary, Adam M. *Antiblack Racism and the AIDS Epidemic: State Intimacies.* New York: Springer, 2014.

Geertz, Clifford. *Local Knowledge: Further Essays in Interpretive Anthropology.* New York: Basic, 1983.

———. *The Religion of Java.* Glencoe, Ill.: Free Press, 1960.

Gell, Alfred. "On Love." *Anthropology of This Century* 2 (October 2011). http://aotcpress.com/articles/love.

Goldman, Robert P. "Fathers, Sons and Gurus: Oedipal Conflict in the Sanskrit Epics." *Journal of Indian Philosophy* 6, no. 4 (1978): 325–92.

———. "Transsexualism, Gender, and Anxiety in Traditional India." *Journal of the American Oriental Society* 113, no. 3 (1993): 374–401.

Goodenough, Ward Hunt. *Property, Kin, and Community on Truk.* New Haven, Conn.: Yale University Press, 1951.

Goodfellow, Aaron. *Gay Fathers, Their Children, and the Making of Kinship.* New York: Fordham University Press, 2015.

———. "Pharmaceutical Intimacy: Sex, Death, and Methamphetamine." *Home Cultures* 5, no. 3 (2008): 271–300.

Greenough, Paul Robert. *Prosperity and Misery in Modern Bengal: The Famine of 1943–1944.* New York: Oxford University Press, 1982.

Guyer, Jane. "The Burden of Wealth and the Lightness of Life: The Body in Body-Decoration in Southern Cameroon." In *Lives in Motion, Indeed: Interdisciplinary Perspectives on Social Change in Honour of Danielle de Lame,* edited by Cristiana Panella. Tervuren: Royal Museum for Central Africa, 2012.

Habib, Mohammad. *Politics and Society during the Early Medieval Period: Collected Works of Professor Mohammad Habib.* Edited by A. K. Nizami. New Delhi: People's Publishing House, 1974.

Hall, Kira. "Intertextual Sexuality." *Journal of Linguistic Anthropology* 15, no. 1 (2005): 125–44.

———. "Unnatural' Gender in Hindi." In *Gender Across Languages: The Linguistic Representation of Women and Men*, edited by Marlis Hellinger and Hadumod Bußmann, 133–62. Amsterdam: John Benjamins, 2002.

Halpern, Richard. *Shakespeare's Perfume: Sodomy and Sublimity in the Sonnets, Wilde, Freud, and Lacan*. Philadelphia: University of Pennsylvania Press, 2002.

Hanif, N. *Biographical Encyclopaedia of Sufis: South Asia*. Vol. 3. New Delhi: Sarup and Sons, 2000.

Hardt, Michael. "For Love or Money." *Cultural Anthropology* 26, no. 4 (2011): 676–82.

Heim, Maria. *"Dana* as a Moral Category." In *Indian Ethics: Classical Traditions and Contemporary Challenges*, edited by Purushottama Bilimoria, Joseph Prabhu, and Renuka M. Sharma, 191–210. Burlington, Vt.: Ashgate, 2007.

Herdt, Gilbert H. *Third Sex, Third Gender: Beyond Sexual Dimorphism in Culture and History*. New York: Zone, 1994.

Hinchy, Jessica. *Governing Gender and Sexuality in Colonial India: The Hijra, c. 1850–1900*. Cambridge and New York: Cambridge University Press, 2019.

———. "Obscenity, Moral Contagion and Masculinity: Hijras in Public Space in Colonial North India." *Asian Studies Review* 38, no. 2 (2014): 274–94.

Holleran, Andrew. *Chronicle of a Plague, Revisited: AIDS and Its Aftermath*. Boston: Da Capo, 2008.

Huberman, Jenny. "The Dangers of Dalālī, the Dangers of Dān." *South Asia: Journal of South Asian Studies* 33, no. 3 (2010): 399–420.

Hudson, Emily T. *Disorienting Dharma: Ethics and the Aesthetics of Suffering in the Mahabharata*. New York: Oxford University Press, 2013.

Jeffrey, Craig. *Timepass: Youth, Class, and the Politics of Waiting in India*. Stanford, Calif.: Stanford University Press, 2010.

Jeffrey, Craig, Patricia Jeffery, and Roger Jeffery. *Degrees without Freedom: Education, Masculinities, and Unemployment in North India*. Stanford, Calif.: Stanford University Press, 2008.

Jurecic, Ann. *Illness as Narrative*. Pittsburgh: University of Pittsburgh Press, 2012.

Khan, Naveeda. "Dogs and Humans and What Earth Can Be: Filaments of Muslim Ecological Thought." *HAU: Journal of Ethnographic Theory* 4, no. 3 (2014): 245–64.

Klot, Jennifer, and Vinh-Kim Nguyen. *The Fourth Wave: Violence, Gender, Culture and HIV in the 21st Century*. Geneva: UNESCO, 2011.

Kockelman, Paul. "From Status to Contract Revisited: Value, Temporality, Circulation and Subjectivity." *Anthropological Theory* 7 (2007): 151–76.

————. "Value Is Life under an Interpretation: Existential Commitments, Instrumental Reasons and Disorienting Metaphors." *Anthropological Theory* 10, no. 1–2 (2010): 149–62.

Lal, Vinay. "Not This, Not That: The Hijras of India and the Cultural Politics of Sexuality." *Social Text* (1999): 119–40.

Lambek, Michael, and Paul Antze, eds. *Illness and Irony: On the Ambiguity of Suffering in Culture.* New York: Berghahn, 2003.

Leach, Edmund Ronald. *Pul Eliya: A Village in Ceylon; A Study of Land Tenure and Kinship.* Cambridge: Cambridge University Press, 1961.

Leung, Helen Hok-Sze. *Farewell My Concubine: A Queer Film Classic.* Vancouver: Arsenal Pulp Press, 2010

————. "Trans on Screen." In *Transgender China*, edited by Howard Chiang, 183–98. New York: Palgrave Macmillan, 2012.

Lewis, Vek. *Crossing Sex and Gender in Latin America.* New York: Palgrave Macmillan, 2010.

Lorway, R., and S. Khan. "Reassembling Epidemiology: Mapping, Monitoring and Making-up People in the Context of HIV Prevention in India." *Social Science and Medicine* 112 (2014): 51–62.

Malinowski, Bronislaw. *Sex and Repression in Savage Society.* Routledge Classics. New York: Routledge, 2001. Originally published in 1927.

Matilal, Bimal Krishna. "The Throne: Was Duryodhana Wrong?" In *The Collected Essays of Bimal Krishna Matlial.* Vol. 2, *Ethics and Epics.* Oxford: Oxford University Press, 2002.

Mattes, Dominik. "Caught in Transition: The Struggle to Live a 'Normal' Life with HIV in Tanzania." *Medical Anthropology* 33, no. 4 (2014): 270–87.

————. "'I Am also a Human Being!' Antiretroviral Treatment in Local Moral Worlds." *Anthropology and Medicine* 19, no. 1 (2012): 75–84.

McClish, Mark, and Patrick Olivelle. *The Arthaśāstra: Selections from the Classic Indian Work on Statecraft.* Indianapolis: Hackett, 2012.

McGuinness, Frank. *In a Town of Five Thousand People.* Loughcrew: Gallery Press, 2012.

McKay, T. "From Marginal to Marginalised: The Inclusion of Men Who Have Sex with Men in Global and National AIDS Programmes and Policy." *Global Public Health* (2016): 1–21. http://doi.org/10.1080/17441692.2016.1143523.

Mehta, Deepak. "Self-Dissolution, Politics and the Work of Affect: The Life and Death of Sufi Baba." *Borderlands* 9, no. 3 (2010).

Mendelsohn, Oliver. "The Pathology of the Indian Legal System." *Modern Asian Studies* 15, no. 4 (1981): 823–63.

Metcalf, Thomas R. *Ideologies of the Raj.* Cambridge University Press, 1997.

Mitchell, Juliet. *Siblings: Sex and Violence.* Cambridge: Polity Press, 2003.

Moon, Michael. *Darger's Resources.* Durham, N.C.: Duke University Press, 2012.

———. "Do You Smoke? Or, Is There Life? After Sex?" In *After Sex?: On Writing since Queer Theory*, edited by Janet Halley and Andrew Parker. Durham, N.C.: Duke University Press, 2011.

Nanda, Serena. *Neither Man nor Woman: The Hijras of India*. Belmont, Calif.: Wadsworth, 1999. Originally published in 1990.

Ochoa, Marcia. *Queen for a Day: Transformistas, Beauty Queens, and the Performance of Femininity in Venezuela*. Durham, N.C.: Duke University Press, 2014.

O'Flaherty, Wendy Doniger. *Siva: The Erotic Ascetic*. Oxford University Press, 1981.

———. *Women, Androgynes, and Other Mythical Beasts*. Chicago: University of Chicago Press, 1982.

Olivelle, Patrick, ed., trans. *Manu's Code of Law: A Critical Edition and Translation of the Manava-Dharmasastra*. Oxford: Oxford University Press, 2004.

Opler, Morris E. "Further Comparative Notes on the Hijarā of India." *American Anthropologist* 63, no. 6 (1961): 1331–32.

———. "The Hijarā (Hermaphrodites) of India and Indian National Character: A Rejoinder." *American Anthropologist* 62, no. 3 (1960): 505–11.

———. "Review of 'The Twice-Born: A Study of a Community of High-Caste Hindus,' by G. Morris Carstairs." *American Anthropologist* 61, no. 1 (1959): 140–42.

Osella, Caroline, and Filippo Osella. *Men and Masculinities in South India*. London: Anthem, 2006.

———. "Vital Exchanges: Land and Persons in Kerala." In *Territory, Soil and Society in the South Asia*, edited by Daniela Berti and Giles Tarabout. New Delhi: Manohar, 2009.

Panchal, Salil. "YK Hamied: Cipla's Fearless Crusader." http://www.forbesindia .com/article/leadership-awards-2016/yk-hamied-ciplas-fearless-crusader /44893/1.

Parry, Jonathan. "The 'Crisis of Corruption' and 'The Idea of India.'" In *Morals of Legitimacy: Between Agency and System*, edited by Italo Pardo, 27–56. New York: Berghahn, 2000.

———. *Death in Banaras*. Cambridge: Cambridge University Press, 1994.

———. "Ghosts, Greed and Sin: The Occupational Identity of the Benares Funeral Priests." *Man* (1980): 88–111.

———. "The Gift, the Indian Gift and the 'Indian Gift.'" *Man* (1986): 453–73.

———. "On the Moral Perils of Exchange." In *Money and the Morality of Exchange*, edited by Jonathan Parry and Maurice Bloch, 64–93. Cambridge: Cambridge University Press, 1989.

Patton, Laurie. *Myth as Argument: The Bṛhaddevatā as Canonical Commentary*. New York: Walter de Gruyter, 1996.

Peletz, Michael G. "Ambivalence in Kinship since the 1940s." In *Relative Values: Reconfiguring Kinship Studies*, edited by Sarah Franklin and Susan McKinnon, 413–44. Durham, N.C.: Duke University Press, 2001.

Pigg, Stacy Leigh. "Expecting the Epidemic: A Social History of the Representation of Sexual Risk in Nepal." *Feminist Media Studies* 2, no. 1 (2002): 97–125.

———. "Globalizing the Facts of Life." In *Sex in Development: Science, Sexuality, and Morality in Global Perspective*, edited by Vincanne Adams and Stacey Leigh Pigg, 39–66. Durham, N.C.: Duke University Press, 2005.

———. "Languages of Sex and AIDS in Nepal: Notes on the Social Production of Commensurability." *Cultural Anthropology* 16, no. 4 (2001): 481–541.

Pinto, Sarah. *Where There Is No Midwife: Birth and Loss in Rural India*. New York: Berghahn, 2008.

Pollock, Sheldon. "The Social Aesthetic and Sanskrit Literary Theory." *Journal of Indian Philosophy* 29, no. 1 (2001): 197–229.

Preston, Laurence W. "A Right to Exist: Eunuchs and the State in Nineteenth-Century India." *Modern Asian Studies* 21, no. 2 (1987): 371–87.

Quignard, Pascal. *Le Sexe et l'Effroi*. Paris: Gallimard, 1994.

Ramanujan, A. K. *The Collected Essays of A. K. Ramanujan*. New Delhi and New York: Oxford University Press, 1999.

Reddy, Gayatri. "'Men' Who Would Be Kings: Celibacy, Emasculation, and the Re-Production of Hijras in Contemporary Indian Politics." *Social Research: An International Quarterly* 70, no. 1 (2003): 163–200.

———. *With Respect to Sex: Negotiating Hijra Identity in South India*. Worlds of Desire. Chicago: University of Chicago Press, 2005.

Robbins, Kenneth X., and John Mcleod. "Cipla's Journey: How a Muslim-Jewish Romance Shaped One of India's Biggest Pharma Firms." https://www.lzb.lt/en/2017/10/13/ciplas-journey-how-a-muslim-jewish-romance-shaped-one-of-indias-biggest-pharma-firms/.

Rocher, Ludo. "'Lawyers' in Classical Hindu Law." *Law and Society Review* (1968): 383–402.

Saria, Vaibhav. "Begging for Change: Hijras, Law and Nationalism." *Contributions to Indian Sociology* 53, no. 1 (2019): 133–57.

———. "The Ungovernable and Dangerous: Children, Sexuality, and Anthropology." In *The Way We Stretch Toward One Another: Thoughts on Anthropology through the Work of Pamela Reynolds*, edited by Todd Meyers, 71–93. Bamenda: African Books Collective, 2017.

Sarkar, Tanika. *Hindu Wife, Hindu Nation: Community, Religion, and Cultural Nationalism*. Bloomington: Indiana University Press, 2001.

Schutz, Alfred. "On Multiple Realities." In *Collected Papers*. Vol. 1, *The Problem of Social Reality*, 207–59. Dordrecht: Springer, 1962.

Sen, Amartya K. *Development as Freedom*. Oxford: Oxford University Press, 2001.

Seremetakis, C. Nadia. *The Last Word: Women, Death, and Divination in Inner Mani*. Chicago: University of Chicago Press, 1991.

Sharma, Pandey Bechan. *Chocolate and Other Writings on Male Homoeroticism*. Translated by Ruth Vanita. Durham, N.C.: Duke University Press, 2009.

Siegel, Lee. *Laughing Matters: Comic Tradition in India*. Chicago: University of Chicago Press, 1987.

Siegel, Lee, and Jayadeva. *Sacred and Profane Dimensions of Love in Indian Traditions as Exemplified in the Gitagovinda of Jayadeva*. Delhi and New York: Oxford University Press, 1978.

Simmel, Georg. *Georg Simmel: On Women, Sexuality, and Love*. Translated by Guy Oakes. New Haven, Conn.: Yale University Press, 1984.

——. "The Sociology of Sociability." *American Journal of Sociology* 55, no. 3 (1949): 254–61.

Singh, Bhrigupati. *Poverty and the Quest for Life: Spiritual and Material Striving in Rural India*. Chicago: University of Chicago Press, 2015.

Skaria, Ajay. "Gandhi's Politics: Liberalism and the Question of the Ashram." *South Atlantic Quarterly* 101, no. 4 (2002): 955–86.

Spivak, Gayatri Chakravorty. "Imperative to Re-Imagine the Planet." In *An Aesthetic Education in the Era of Globalization*. Cambridge, Mass.: Harvard University Press, 2012.

Staples, James. "Begging Questions: Leprosy and Alms Collection in Mumbai." In *Livelihoods at the Margins: Surviving the City*, edited by James Staples. Walnut Creek, Calif.: Left Coast, 2007.

——. "Disguise, Revelation and Copyright: Disassembling the South Indian Leper." *Journal of the Royal Anthropological Institute* 9, no. 2 (2003): 295–315.

Stevenson, Lisa. *Life beside Itself: Imagining Care in the Canadian Arctic*. Berkeley: University of California Press, 2014.

Thapar, Romila. "Genealogical Patterns as Perceptions of the Past." *Studies in History* 7, no. 1 (1991): 1–36.

——. "Sacrifice, Surplus, and the Soul." *History of Religions* 33, no. 4 (1994): 305–24.

Thomann, M. "HIV Vulnerability and the Erasure of Sexual and Gender Diversity in Abidjan, Côte d'Ivoire." *Global Public Health* (2016): 1–16. http://doi.org/10.1080/17441692.2016.1143524.

Thomas, Lynn. "Parasurama and Time." In *Myth and Mythmaking: Continuous Evolution in Indian Tradition*, edited by Julia Leslie. Surrey: Curzon, 1996.

Towle, Evan B., and Lynn Marie Morgan. "Romancing the Transgender Native: Rethinking the Use of the 'Third Gender' Concept." *GLQ: A Journal of Lesbian and Gay Studies* 8, no. 4 (2002): 469–97.

Trautmann, Thomas R. *Arthashastra: The Science of Wealth*. New Delhi: Allen Lane Penguin Books India, 2012.

Trawick, Margaret. *Notes on Love in a Tamil Family*. Berkeley: University of California Press, 1992.

Upadhyay, Nishant, and Sandeep Bakshi. "Translating Queer: Reading Caste, Decolonizing Praxis." In *The Routledge Handbook of Translation, Feminism and Gender*, edited by Luise von Flotow and Hala Kamal. London and New York: Routledge, 2020.

Vyas, M. D., and Yogesh Shingala. *The Life Style of the Eunuchs*. New Delhi: Anmol, 1987.

Vyāsa. *The Mahabharata*. Vol. 2, Book 2: *The Book of Assembly*; Book 3: *The Book of the Forest*. Translated by J. A. B. van Buitenen. Chicago: University of Chicago Press, 1981.

——. *Mahābhārata: Preparations for War*. Book 5, Vol. 1; Vol. 2: Translated by Kathleen Garbutt. Clay Sanskrit Library. New York University Press, 2008.

Weheliye, Alexander. *Habeas Viscus: Racializing Assemblages, Biopolitics, and Black Feminist Theories of the Human*. Durham, N.C.: Duke University Press, 2014.

Weightman, Simon. "The Symmetry of *Madhumalati*." In *Madhumalati: An Indian Sufi Romance*. Translated by Aditya Behl. New York: Oxford University Press, 2001.

Weston, Kath. *Families We Choose: Lesbians, Gays, Kinship*. New York: Columbia University Press, 1991.

White, David Gordon. *Kiss of the Yogini: 'Tantric Sex' in Its South Asian Contexts*. Chicago: University of Chicago Press, 2003.

White, E., ed. *Loss within Loss: Artists in the Age of AIDS*. Madison: University of Wisconsin Press, 2002.

Woodroffe, Sir John. *Introduction to Tantra Sastra*. 5th ed. Madras, 1969.

Zimman, Lal, and Kira Hall. "Language, Embodiment, and the 'Third Sex.'" In *Language and Identities*, edited by Carmen Llamas and Dominic Watt, 166–78. Edinburgh: Edinburgh University Press, 2010.

Zimmermann, Francis. "The Love-Lorn Consumptive: South Asian Ethnography and the Psychosomatic Paradigm." *Anthropologies of Medicine* 7 (1991): 185–95.

INDEX

medications, HIV, 181, 190, 194–95
Mendelsohn, Oliver, 69–70, 211nn9,11
men who have sex with men (MSM),
  23, 183, 185–86, 191–93
milk, 218n10
miscarriage, 209n37
Mitchell, Juliet, 212n13
monks, 120
Moon, Michael, 149, 154–57
mothers, 32, 40, 45, 67, 80, 85–86, 159, 162
"Mourning and Melancholia" (Freud),
  94–95
munis, 120–21

Nanda, Serena, 19, 161, 164, 166, 175–76,
  206n10, 225n59
nationalism, 4, 15, 202n8, 223n38
No Aging in India (Cohen), 79–80
nocturnal emissions, 150–51
*No Future: Queer Theory and the Death
  Drive* (Edelman), 5–6
noncruelty, 103, 124, 127–28
nonviolence, 103, 127

Oedipus, 158–59
old age, 79–80, 89–90, 94
Olivelle, Patrick, 135
"On the Moral Perils of Exchange"
  (Parry), 112–13
Opler, Morris E., 103, 105
Osella, Caroline, 151
Osella, Filippo, 151

Packard, Randall, 193–94
pain, 54–59
Parry, Jonathan, 112–113, 115, 131, 219n9
pedagogy, 30–31, 142–49, 155
Pedagogy and Pederasty (Bersani),
  148–49
pederasty, 143–44, 148–49
Pehchan program, 182–83

penetration, 18, 142–46, 148–49, 155
performance, 26, 42, 64, 111, 201n5
perfume, 8–9
physical space, 56–57
play, 133–34, 142–49
"Pleasures of Castration, The: The
  Postoperative Status of Hijras,
  Jankhas, and Academics" (Cohen),
  101–2
political pornography, 12
political theology, 2, 6
politicians, 128–32, 138
Pollock, Sheldon, 52–55, 57
pornography, political, 12
poverty, 3, 14, 61, 84, 133, 179, 193–94, 196
pregnancy, 11, 33–42, 45, 47, 61
presents, 166–68
priests, 219n9, 220n22
property taxes, 67, 210n4
property transmission, 68–70, 80–81,
  212n17
prostitution. *See* sex work
psychoanalytic theory, 2–3, 19, 158
punishment, 144–45, 157

queer theory, 2, 5–7

Ram (or Rama), 84, 136
Rao, P. V. Narasimha, 129
rape, 142. *See also* violence
rasa, 50–55
Reddy, Gayatri, 19, 40, 42, 123, 147–148,
  164–67, 175, 206n10, 225n59, 229n58
renaming, 4
rent collection, 221n34
reproductive futurism, 6–7
ritual labor, 116, 133

sadaa suhaagan, 39, 43–44, 56, 208n19
sadism/masochism (S/M), 189
sangha, 102, 217n6, 231n15

Vaibhav Saria is Assistant Professor of Gender, Sexuality, and Women's Studies at Simon Fraser University.